Foundations and Diseases of Circulatory System

循环系统基础与疾病

Editor-in-Chief of the Book/主编

Wang Yuchun/王玉春

Deputy Editors-in-Chief of the Book/副主编

Jin Haifeng/金海峰　　Yang Hongyan/杨宏艳

Sandeep Shrestha/桑迪普·什雷斯塔

科 学 出 版 社

北 京

内 容 简 介

本教材是"基础医学课程整合系列教材"的一个分册，遵循"以器官系统为中心"的国际医学教育模式，按照课程改革要求，根据历年来华留学生的实际情况，为开展英语教学而策划编写的实用教材。本教材整合了系统解剖学、组织胚胎学、生理学、病理学、病理生理学及药理学等基础医学课程中与循环系统相关的知识内容，涵盖循环系统的解剖与组织结构、生理功能、病理变化、疾病的病理生理机制及药物治疗等知识点。在编写过程中注重打破学科间壁垒，删除学科间重复知识点，并增加章节小结及关键词的中英文注解等，为学生学习循环系统医学知识提供一个系统、完整的内容体系。

本教材适用于各层次的医学生，同时也为双语教学或留学生教学的教师提供参考。

图书在版编目（CIP）数据

循环系统基础与疾病=Foundations and Diseases of Circulatory System：英文/王玉春主编. —北京：科学出版社，2024.3
ISBN 978-7-03-078330-1

Ⅰ.①循… Ⅱ.①王… Ⅲ.①心脏血管疾病–诊疗–英文 Ⅳ.① R54

中国国家版本馆 CIP 数据核字（2024）第 064063 号

责任编辑：朱　华/责任校对：宁辉彩
责任印制：张　伟/封面设计：陈　敬

科 学 出 版 社 出版
北京东黄城根北街 16 号
邮政编码：100717
http://www.sciencep.com

涿州市般润文化传播有限公司印刷
科学出版社发行　各地新华书店经销
*

2024 年 3 月第 一 版　开本：787×1092　1/16
2024 年 3 月第一次印刷　印张：8
字数：290 000

定价：88.00 元
（如有印装质量问题，我社负责调换）

编　委　会
Editorial Committee

General Foreword

With the rapid development of international medical education in China, more and more international medical students are studying in China. The teaching mode adopted by colleges and universities for international medical students in China is crucial for the quality of international physicians trained in China. The medical teaching mode with "organ system as the center" is the prevailing trend in the development of international medical education. The integrated teaching materials for Chinese medical undergraduates are close to saturation, while reformation and development of integrated teaching materials for international medical undergraduates are relatively lagging behind. The series of integrated basic medical textbooks are planned and written in response to the trend of reform in international medical education model and to the needs of education of international students. They enrich the English teaching resources and promote the pace of the teaching reform for international students in China, which has far-reaching significance for the development of medical education.

This series of textbooks is written by teachers who have been working at the forefront of teaching and scientific research for a long time. They come from the teaching departments of Qiqihar Medical University, Shantou University Medical College, and Shenyang Medical College, most of whom have rich teaching experience with international students. They strive for systematic, innovative, and well-written content. This series of textbooks includes four volumes, *Foundations and Diseases of Locomotor System, Foundations and Diseases of Circulatory System, Foundations and Diseases of Nervous System, Foundations and Diseases of Splanchnology*, which are scheduled for publication. Each volume is arranged overall with the concept of "organ system integration", organically integrated with the anatomy of each system structural organisation, physiological functions, pathological changes, the pathophysiology of disease and medication to form "a series of integrated medical textbooks (English edition) based on the human organs". In the process of writing, we intend to break the barriers and delete repetitive knowledge between disciplines, and increase the chapter summary and annotation of keywords in both Chinese and English to provide a systematic and complete teaching design and content system for students to learn medical knowledge. They are suitable for international medical students, undergraduates and postgraduates, also serve as a good reference book for clinical teachers and clinical medical staff.

In the course of planning and writing the textbook, we were greatly supported and helped by leaders of Qiqihar Medical University. Here, we would like to express our heartfelt thanks to them. The content and format of this book is a new attempt. We invite readers and colleagues to provide feedback if there are any deficiencies.

Li Tao, Wang Yuchun
March 2023

序

随着我国医学教育事业的蓬勃发展，来华的医学专业留学生越来越多，高校对来华医学留学生采用的授课模式关乎我国培养国际医师的质量。"以器官系统为中心"的医学教学模式是国际医学教育发展的总趋势，我国本科医学生的课程整合教材已接近饱和，而针对来华医学本科留学生的课程整合改革发展却相对滞后。本基础医学课程整合系列教材顺应我国国际医学教育改革趋势，配合留学生教学需求，在丰富留学生教学资源的同时，推动了我国医学留学生教学改革的步伐，对医学教育的发展具有深远意义。

本系列教材由长期工作在教学和科研一线的教师编写而成，他们来自齐齐哈尔医学院、汕头大学医学院及沈阳医学院等教学单位，具有丰富的留学生教学经验；在编写宗旨上力求体系统一、理念创新及编写精美。全套书四册，包括《运动系统基础与疾病》《循环系统基础与疾病》《神经系统基础与疾病》《内脏系统基础与疾病》，计划陆续出版。每册书按照"器官系统整合"的理念，统筹安排教材内容，将各系统的解剖与组织结构、生理功能、病理变化、疾病的病理生理机制和药物治疗等有机融合，形成"以人体器官系统为基础的医学整合系列教材（英文版）"。本书在编写过程中注重打破学科间壁垒，删除学科间重复知识点，并增加章节小结、关键词的中英文注解等，为学生学习医学知识提供一个系统、完整的内容体系，适用于医学留学生与医学本科生、研究生，也是临床专业教师、临床医务工作者良好的参考用书。

本教材在编写过程中得到了齐齐哈尔医学院领导的支持和帮助，在此表示由衷的感谢。本书的内容和形式是一次全新的尝试，有不完善之处，敬请各位读者和同行不吝指教！

李 涛 王玉春

2023年3月

Preface

Foundations and Diseases of Circulatory System is a part of the series of integrated medical textbooks based on the human organ system, organized and written by the Qiqihar Medical University and Shantou University Medical College. It is a basic medical teaching material planned and written in response to the trend of reform on international medical education model with "organ system as the center" and to the needs of education of international students.

The book integrates knowledge related to the circulatory system in anatomy, physiology, pathology, pathophysiology, pharmacology, system histology and embryology and other basic medical courses. The content covers anatomy and histology, physiological functions, pathological changes, the pathophysiology of diseases, and drug treatment. In the process of writing, we intend to break the barriers and delete repetitive knowledge between disciplines, and increase the chapter summary and annotation of keywords in both Chinese and English to provide a systematic complete teaching design and content system for students to learn medical knowledge. This textbook is suitable for medical students at all levels, and also provides reference for bilingual teaching or teaching international students.

In the course of planning and writing the textbook, we were greatly supported and helped by many teachers in the departments of anatomy, histology and embryology, physiology, pathology and pharmacology of Qiqihar Medical University. Here, we would like to express our heartfelt gratitude to the above staff for their contributions.

Due to the limitation of the editors' level, readers and colleagues are invited to provide feedback and comments on any deficiency.

Wang Yuchun
March 2023

前　言

　　《循环系统基础与疾病》是由齐齐哈尔医学院作为主要编写单位,并联合汕头大学医学院编写的基础医学课程整合系列教材的一部分,是顺应"以器官系统为中心"的国际医学教育模式改革趋势,适应留学生教学需求而策划编写的系列医学基础课程教材。

　　《循环系统基础与疾病》教材整合了生理学、病理学、病理生理学、药理学、系统解剖学以及组织胚胎学等基础医学课程中与循环系统相关的知识内容,内容涵盖循环系统的解剖与组织结构、生理功能、病理变化、疾病的病理生理机制及药物治疗。在编写过程中注重打破学科间壁垒,删除学科间重复知识点,并增加章节小结、关键词的中英文注解等,为学生学习医学知识提供一个系统、完整的内容体系,既适用于各层次的医学生,又为双语教学或留学生教学的教师提供参考。

　　在教材的规划和编写过程中,本教材得到了齐齐哈尔医学院解剖学、组织胚胎学、生理学、病理学、病理生理学和药理学等多个教研室多位教师的大力支持和无私帮助,在此对以上人员的付出和劳动,表示由衷的感谢。

　　限于编者的水平,不完善之处,敬请各位读者和同行不吝指教!

王玉春

2023年3月

Contents

Part Ⅰ   Anatomical Structure of Circulatory System

Part Ⅱ   Cardiovascular Histology

Part Ⅲ   Cardiovascular Physiology

Part Ⅳ   Pathologic Circulatory System

Part Ⅴ   Cardiovascular Pathophysiology

Part VI Drugs Affecting the Circulatory System

Part Ⅰ　Anatomical Structure of Circulatory System

Chapter 1　General Description

The cardiovascular system includes the **heart** (心脏), **arteries** (动脉), **veins** (静脉) and **capillaries** (毛细血管).

1.1　Heart

As the central organ of the cardiovascular system, the heart function is similar to the power pump. It is responsible for connecting arteries and veins, and is mainly composed of myocardium. Besides it also has certain endocrine functions. The heart is divided into right and left halves by the septum. Each half contains two chambers, and the heart has four chambers in total. The upper two chambers are called the **right and left atria** (心房). Their main function is to receive the blood from the veins and transfer it to the **ventricles** (心室). The lower two chambers are called the right and left ventricles, and the main function of the ventricles is to pump the blood into arteries. The ipsilateral atrium and ventricle are connected with each other by the atrioventricular orifice. The part of the heart septum between the two atria is called the **interatrial septum** (房间隔), and the part of heart septum between the two ventricles is called the **interventricular septum** (室间隔). The atrium are always connected to the veins, while the ventricles are connected to the arteries. The valves are located on the atrioventricular orifice and ostia of the arteries. Their function is to ensure proper blood flow in the correct direction through the heart.

1.2　Artery

These are the vessels that carry blood away from the heart. The wall of the artery is thicker than that of the veins, and includes 3 layers. The inner layer is thin and rich in endothelial cells, which can reduce the blood flow resistance. The middle layer is thicker than the inner layer, rich in collagenous fibers and elastic fibers, which can stimulate the circulation of blood. The outer layer is mainly composed of loose connective tissue, which can prevent the over expansion of ventricle. The arteries can be classified into 3 types based on their origin and size. They are the large arteries, medium arteries, and arterioles. Corresponding to the characteristics of the arterial wall, the large artery is also called the **elastic artery** (弹性动脉); the medium artery is also called the **muscular artery** (肌性动脉). The diameter of arteriole is just about 0.3mm–1mm and visible to the naked eye. The arteries are constantly branching in the course and the branches become more and more, eventually forming capillaries.

1.3　Capillary

There are a lot of capillaries found in various tissues and organs, except for the cornea, lens, cartilage, hairs, and so on, forming an anastomosing network. The capillary is thin, with high permeability, and the blood flow in the tube is slow. It is the place of material exchange between the blood and the tissue fluid.

1.4　Vein

Veins are the vessels that transfer blood back into the heart. The small veins are usually formed by the confluence of capillaries. The tributaries are continuously accepted during the process of small vein confluence, finally forming the middle vein or large vein. The walls of the veins also contain three layers of membrane, but the boundary is not obvious. Compared with those of the artery, the walls of the vein are thin, with large lumen, less elasticity, and high volume of blood.

There are two types of blood circulation patterns in the human body. In the **systemic circulation** (体循环), the blood is pumped out from the left ventricle, and supplies blood to the entire body through the aorta and its branches. The blood is exchanged with the surrounding tissues and cells for substances and gases, and then returns to the right atrium through veins. In the **pulmonary circulation** (肺循环), the blood is pumped from the right ventricle, and then reaches the alveolar capillary through the pulmonary trunk and its branches for gaseous exchange. It finally enters the left atrium through the pulmonary veins. The systemic circulation and the pulmonary circulation are carried out simultaneously. The long circulation of systemic circulation passes through a wide range, nourishing the whole body with arterial blood, and transporting the whole body's metabolites and carbon dioxide to the heart. The pulmonary circulation is short, only through the lungs, which mainly changes the venous blood into oxygen-saturated arterial blood.

1.5 Vascular Anastomoses

In addition to arterial-capillary-venous connections, the vascular anastomoses also include **arterial anastomoses** (动脉间吻合), **venous anastomoses** (静脉间吻合), **arteriovenous anastomoses** (动静脉吻合), and **collateral anastomoses** (侧支吻合).

1.5.1 Arterial Anastomoses

The two arteries of different parts or organs in the body can be connected by a traffic branch. In the parts of frequent movement, the branches of adjacent arteries often form **arterial rete** (动脉网), like the arterial rete of the elbow joint. The endings or branches of adjacent arteries can also form an **arterial arch** (动脉弓), like the superficial palmar arch. These anastomoses can shorten the time of blood circulation and regulate blood flow.

1.5.2 Venous Anastomoses

The venous anastomoses are similar to the arterial

anastomoses, but are more in number than the arterial anastomoses. The veins usually surround the organs or are within the walls of the organs and form the **venous plexus** (静脉丛), which ensure that the blood flow is unobstructed when the viscera is enlarged or the wall of the cavity is pressed.

1.5.3 Arteriovenous Anastomoses

In many places of the body, some small arteries can communicate directly with small veins, like ones in the terminal phalanges, nose, skin of external ear, lip, and so on. This anastomosis can regulate local blood flow and body temperature.

1.5.4 Collateral Anastomoses

Some vascular trunks send out many collateral branches at different heights, and these branches go parallel with the trunk forming the collateral anastomoses. In the pathological conditions, if the trunk is blocked, the collateral anastomoses can maintain the blood supply, which have great significance for the blood circulation.

Summary

本章简要概述了心血管系统的组成和血管间的吻合。

心血管系统是由心脏、动脉、毛细血管和静脉组成。血液由左心室泵出，经主动脉及其分支到达全身毛细血管，血液在此与周围的组织、细胞进行物质和气体交换，再通过各级静脉，最后经上、下腔静脉及心冠状窦返回右心房，这一循环称为体循环。肺循环是血液由右心室搏出，经肺动脉干及其各级分支到达肺泡毛细血管进行气体交换，再经肺静脉进入左心房。

人体的血管除动脉-毛细血管-静脉相通连外，动脉与动脉之间，静脉与静脉之间甚至动脉与静脉之间，可借血管支彼此连结，形成血管吻合。

学生应重点学习心血管系统的组成，体循环和肺循环的途径，掌握了解血管吻合及其功能意义。

Zhang Shanqiang, Wang Lulu (张善强、王璐璐)

Chapter 2　Heart

2.1　Position, Shape and Adjacent Structures

The heart is a hollow muscular organ with a shape of an inverted and slightly flattened cone. It is surrounded by the pericardium which is obliquely located in the middle mediastinum of the thoracic cavity. In China, an average adult heart is 284±50(g) in males and 258±49(g) in females. However, the weight of the heart can vary depending on age, body weight, and physical activity.

About 2/3 of the heart is located on the left side of the median line, and 1/3 on the right side (Fig. 2-1). In front of the heart, there is the body of sternum and the second to sixth costal cartilages. The fifth to eighth vertebrae are located behind the heart. On the

two lateral sides, the heart is close to the pleural cavity and lungs. Above the heart, there are large blood vessels which enter and exit the heart. The diaphragm is located below the heart. A 45° angle is formed by the median line of the body and the long axis of the heart from the right shoulder obliquely to the left subcostal region.

In rare cases, the heart can appear in the opposite position, and usually concomitant with the reversal of the visceral organs in the abdominal cavity.

The heart includes an apex, a base, two surfaces, three borders, and four grooves on the surface (Fig. 2-2, Fig. 2-3).

The **cardiac apex** (心尖) is blunt and round, formed by the left ventricle and located close to the left anterior chest wall. The cardiac apex faces the left anterior and mild downward direction. On the medial side of the midclavicular line, about 1–2 centimeters inner, the apical pulsation is auscultated at the left fifth intercostal space.

The **cardiac base** (心底) faces right posterior direction and is formed by the left and right atria. The superior and inferior vena cava are connected to the right atrium. The left and right pulmonary veins are connected to the left atrium. Behind the cardiac base, there are esophagus, aorta, and vagus nerve.

The **sternocostal surface** (胸肋面) is also called the **anterior surface** (前面). It is formed mainly by the right atrium and right ventricle, and partly by the left auricle and left ventricle.

In addition to the pericardium, most of this surface is covered by the pleuras and lungs, and the small part is adjacent to the lower part of the sternal body and the 4th to 6th costal cartilages on the left. So the

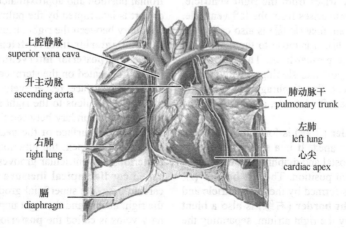

Figure 2-1　Position of the heart.

上腔静脉
superior vena cava

升主动脉
ascending aorta

右肺
right lung

膈
diaphragm

肺动脉干
pulmonary trunk

左肺
left lung

心尖
cardiac apex

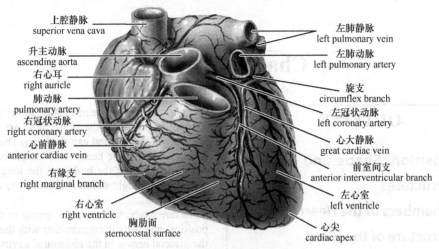

上腔静脉
superior vena cava

升主动脉
ascending aorta

右心耳
right auricle

肺动脉
pulmonary artery

右冠状动脉
right coronary artery

心前静脉
anterior cardiac vein

右缘支
right marginal branch

右心室
right ventricle

胸肋面
sternocostal surface

左肺静脉
left pulmonary vein

左肺动脉
left pulmonary artery

旋支
circumflex branch

左冠状动脉
left coronary artery

心大静脉
great cardiac vein

前室间支
anterior interventricular branch

左心室
left ventricle

心尖
cardiac apex

Figure 2-2　External features and vessels of the heart (anterior view).

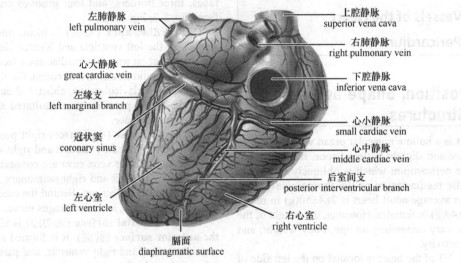

左肺静脉
left pulmonary vein

心大静脉
great cardiac vein

左缘支
left marginal branch

冠状窦
coronary sinus

左心室
left ventricle

上腔静脉
superior vena cava

右肺静脉
right pulmonary vein

下腔静脉
inferior vena cava

心小静脉
small cardiac vein

心中静脉
middle cardiac vein

后室间支
posterior interventricular branch

右心室
right ventricle

膈面
diaphragmatic surface

Figure 2-3　External features and vessels of the heart (posterior view).

intracardiac injections are to be given at the level of the left 4th intercostal space and the left margin of the sternum. In the upper part of the sternocostal surface, the pulmonary trunk arises from the right ventricle, and the ascending aorta arises from the left ventricle. The **diaphragmatic surface** (膈面) is also called the **inferior surface** (下面). It is close to the diaphragm and separated by the pericardium. This surface is almost in horizontal position, sloping downward and slightly toward the rear. The diaphragmatic surface is formed mainly by the left ventricle, and partly by the right ventricle.

　　The **inferior border** (下缘) is formed by the right ventricle and cardiac apex. It is a sharp border that separates the sternocostal and diaphragmatic surfaces, almost in a horizontal position. The **left border** (左缘) is blunt, which is formed by the left ventricle and left auricle. The **right border** (右缘) is also a blunt border and formed by the right atrium, separating the sternocostal and cardiac base.

　　There are four grooves on the surface of the heart, which serve as demarcations of the four heart chambers. The **coronary sulcus** (冠状沟) is almost in frontal position and approximately circular. Its anterior part is interrupted by the pulmonary trunk. It is the boundary between the right atrium and the left ventricle. The **anterior interventricular groove** (前室间沟) and the **posterior interventricular groove** (后室间沟) are located on the sternocostal surface and diaphragmatic surface, respectively. Their course is from the coronary sulcus to the right side of cardiac apex, forming the boundary between the left and right ventricles on the surface of the heart. On the right side of the cardiac apex, the junction of the anterior and posterior interventricular grooves is sunken, which is called **cardiac apical incisure** (心尖切迹). On the cardiac base, the superficial groove at the junction of the right atrium and the right upper and lower pulmonary veins is called the **posterior interatrial groove** (后房间沟), which is the boundary between the left and right atria. The junction of coronary sulcus, posterior interventricular groove and posterior interatrial groove is called the crux of the heart, which is an important landmark of the heart's surface. In its depths, there are some important blood vessels and nerves.

2.2　Chambers of the Heart

2.2.1　Right Atrium

The **right atrium** (右心房) (Fig. 2-4) is located in the right upper part of the heart with a large cavity and thin wall, which can be divided into the anterior and posterior parts. The anterior part is called the **atrium proper** (固有心房), while the posterior part

is called the **sinus venarum cavarum** (腔静脉窦). The boundary between these two parts is called the **sulcus terminalis** (界沟), which is the vertical sulcus located between the anterior borders of the superior and inferior vena cava. It corresponds internally to the **crista terminalis** (界嵴).

2.2.1.1　Atrium proper

The atrium proper is the anterior part of the right atrium. On its inner surface, there are many rough parallel arrangements of muscle bundles, called the **pectinate muscles** (梳状肌). These muscles originate from the crista terminalis and extend anterolaterally towards the right atrioventricular orifice. The atrial wall between the pectinate muscles is thin, and the pectinate muscles are interlaced with each other to form a network at the point of auricle.

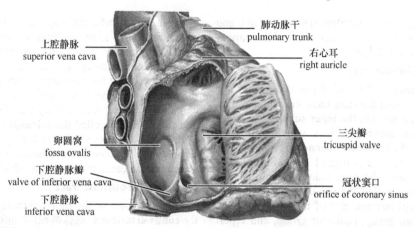

上腔静脉　superior vena cava
肺动脉干　pulmonary trunk
右心耳　right auricle
卵圆窝　fossa ovalis
下腔静脉瓣　valve of inferior vena cava
下腔静脉　inferior vena cava
三尖瓣　tricuspid valve
冠状窦口　orifice of coronary sinus

Figure 2-4　Right atrium.

2.2.1.2　Sinus venarum cavarum

The inner surface of sinus venarum cavarum is smooth. The **orifice of superior vena cava** (上腔静脉口) is opening in the upper part of right atrium, and the **orifice of inferior vena cava** (下腔静脉口) is opening in the lower part of right atrium. Of these two orifices, the superior vena cava usually has no valve, and the **valve of inferior vena cava** (Eustachian valve, 下腔静脉瓣) is located on the anterior border of the orifice.

The **orifice of coronary sinus** (冠状窦口) is located between the orifice of inferior vena cava and the right atrioventricular orifice. The **valve of coronary sinus** (冠状窦瓣) is located on the posterior border of the orifice of the coronary sinus, with an occurrence rate of 70%.

The posterior part of right atrial medial wall is formed mainly by interatrial septum. The **fossa ovalis** (卵圆窝) is a shallow depression located on the lower-central part of right atrial median wall. The fossa ovalis is the remnant of the closure of the foramen ovale during the embryonic period. Therefore, it is relatively weak.

Between the anteromedial orifice of coronary sinus, the septal leaflet of the tricuspid valve, and the **Todaro tendon** (托达罗腱), there is an area called **Koch triangle** (科赫三角). The Todaro tendon is a tendinous structure below the endocardium which is anterior to the orifice of inferior vena cava. It is attached to the central fibrous body through the atrial septum and extends back to the valve of inferior vena cava. The atrioventricular node is located within the Koch triangle.

2.2.2　Right Ventricle

The **right ventricle** (右心室) (Fig. 2-5) is located on the anteroinferior side of the right atrium. It lies behind the left border of sternum and 4–5 costal cartilage. The anterior wall of the right ventricle is near the thorax, just located between the right coronary sulcus, anterior interventricular groove, right border of the heart, and the orifice of pulmonary artery. Majority of the sternocostal surface is formed by the right ventricle. The wall of the right ventricle is thin and only 1/3 of the thickness of the left ventricular wall.

The right ventricle can be divided into the **inflow**

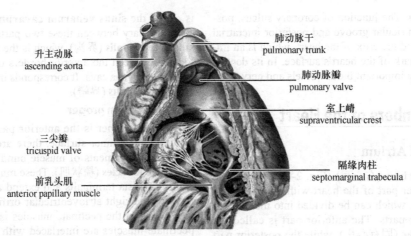

升主动脉
ascending aorta

肺动脉干
pulmonary trunk

肺动脉瓣
pulmonary valve

室上嵴
supraventricular crest

三尖瓣
tricuspid valve

隔缘肉柱
septomarginal trabecula

前乳头肌
anterior papillary muscle

Figure 2-5　Right ventricle.

tract (流入道) and the **outflow tract** (流出道), and the boundary of these two tracts is called the **supra-ventricular crest** (室上嵴).

2.2.2.1　The inflow tract

The inflow tract is also called the **sinus part** (窦部). It extends from the right atrioventricular orifice to the cardiac apex. On the inner surface, there are many interlaced muscular ridges, which are known collectively as the **trabeculae carneae** (肉柱). There-fore, the inner surface is rugged. In addition to the trabeculae carneae, there are many pyramid shaped muscular ridges called the **papillary muscles** (乳头肌). The papillary muscles of the right ventricle include anterior group, posterior group, and septal group. The anterior group contains 1–5 **anterior papillary muscles** (前乳头肌), which are located on the lower-middle part of the anterior ventricular wall. The posterior group includes 2–3 **posterior papillary muscles** (后乳头肌), which are located on the inferi-or ventricular wall. The **septal papillary muscles** (隔侧乳头肌) are on the right side of the upper-middle part of the interventricular septum. In the root of the anterior papillary muscles, there is a muscular bundle crossing from the ventricular cavity to the lower parts of the interventricular septum, which forms the lower boundary of the inflow tract. This muscular bundle is called the **septomarginal trabecula** (隔缘肉柱), and it is also termed the **moderator band** (节制索), which has the function of preventing overexpansion of the ventricle.

The entrance of the inflow tract is an oval opening called the **right atrioventricular orifice** (右房室口). Around the orifice, there is a dense connective tissue called the **tricuspid annulus** (三尖瓣环). The tricuspid valves are three approximately triangular leaflets, and the bases of the valves are attached to the annulus. The apexes of the valves are free and droop-ing into the ventricular cavity. Based on the location, the three leaflets are named as **anterior cusp** (前尖), **posterior cusp** (后尖), and the **septal cusp** (隔侧尖).

Between the two adjacent cusps, the connective tissues can be referred to as anteroseptal commissure, postero-medial commissure, and antero-posterior commissure. **Chordae tendineae** (腱索) are the tendinous struc-tures that connect the papillary muscles to the tricus-pid valves. The tricuspid annulus, tricuspid valves, chordae tendineae, and papillary muscles, in structure and function, are called the **tricuspid complex** (三尖瓣复合体). These structures jointly guarantee the one-way flow of blood. Alterations of anyone in these structures can cause tricuspid valve dysfunction.

2.2.2.2　The outflow tract

The outflow tract of the right ventricle is also called the **conus arteriosus** (动脉圆锥) or infundibular part. The outflow tract is cone-shaped, and the inner sur-face is smooth. On the upper end of the outflow tract, the right ventricle is connected to the pulmonary trunk through the orifice of pulmonary trunk. On the orifice of pulmonary trunk, there are three semilunar fibrous rings connected with each other, and these rings are collectively referred to as **annulus of pulmonary valve** (肺动脉瓣环). The **pulmonary valve** (肺动脉瓣) is formed by three semilunar-shaped valves that are attached to the annulus. The free margins of the valves face towards the direction of the pulmonary trunk, and the central thickening of the free margin of each valve is called **nodule of the semilunar valve** (半月瓣小结). The space between each valve and the corresponding wall of the pulmonary trunk is called **sinus of pulmonary trunk** (肺动脉窦). The main function of the pulmonary valves is to prevent the backflow of blood into the right ventricle.

2.2.3　Left Atrium

The **left atrium** (左心房) is located on the left rear direction of the right atrium, which forms the large part of the cardiac base. The left atrium is posterior to the ascending aorta and pulmonary trunk, and anterior to the esophagus. The left atrium can be divided into the **left auricle** (左心耳) and the **atrium proper** (固有心房), according to the development of the embryo.

2.2.3.1　Left auricle

The left auricle is narrower and longer than the right auricle, and there are some notches on the border. The inner surface also has the pectinate muscles, but the distribution is uneven. Compared with the right auricle, the pectinate muscles of the left auricle are not well developed.

2.2.3.2　Atrium proper

The inner surface of the atrium proper is smooth, and there are four openings on the two lateral sides of the posterior wall to communicate with the left and right pulmonary veins. The orifices of the pulmonary veins have no valves, but the atrial muscle extending from the left atrial wall around the pulmonary veins for 1–2 centimeters may play the role of a sphincter. The left atrium is connected with the left ventricle by the **left atrioventricular orifice** (左房室口).

2.2.4　Left Ventricle

The **left ventricle** (左心室) is a cone-shaped cavity that is located on the left rear direction of the right ventricle. The left ventricle can be divided into the inflow tract and outflow tract by the anterior leaflet of the mitral valve.

2.2.4.1　The inflow tract

The inflow tract is also called the sinus part, which is located on the left rear direction of the anterior leaflet of the mitral valve. The entrance of the left ventricular inflow tract is through the left atrioventricular orifice. The dense connective tissue around the orifice is **mitral annulus** (二尖瓣环). The base of mitral valve (**left atrioventricular valve**, 左房室瓣) is attached to the annulus. The mitral annulus can be divided into the **anterior cusp** (前尖) and the **posterior cusp** (后尖) by the two deep notches.

The inflow tract of the left ventricle also has the papillary muscles, including the **anterior papillary muscle** (前乳头肌) and **posterior papillary muscle** (后乳头肌). These papillary muscles supply the chordae tendineae to both the leaflets of the mitral valve. The **mitral complex** (二尖瓣复合体) is composed of the mitral annulus, mitral valves, papillary muscles, and the chordae tendineae. The functions of the mitral complex are similar to that of the tricuspid complex, although the components are slightly different.

2.2.4.2　The outflow tract

The outflow tract of left ventricle is also named the **aortic vestibule** (主动脉前庭). The wall of the outflow tract is smooth, and it is formed by the upper part of the interventricular septum and anterior cusp of the mitral valve. The upper boundary of the outflow tract is the **aortic orifice** (主动脉口). On the

orifice, there is a fibrous ring called the **annulus of aortic valve** (主动脉瓣环), and the aortic valves are attached to the annulus. The aortic valves consist of three semilunar shaped valves. Based on the location, the valves they can be referred as the left, right and posterior valve. The space between each valve and the corresponding wall is knowns as the aortic sinus. The left and right coronary arteries originate from the wall of the left and right aortic sinuses, respectively.

2.3　Structure of the Heart

2.3.1　Fibrous Skeleton of the Heart

The **fibrous skeleton of heart** (心纤维性支架) is also called the fibrous framework. It is located around the atrioventricular orifice, the orifice of pulmonary trunk, and the aortic orifice, which are formed by dense connective tissue. The fibrous skeleton of the heart is tough and elastic, which provides attachment points for cardiac muscle fibers and heart valves. It plays a supportive and stabilizing role in cardiac muscle movement.

The fibrous skeleton of the heart consists of two fibrous trigones, four fibrous annuli, and the membranous part of the interventricular septum and so on (Fig. 2-6).

The **right fibrous trigone** (右纤维三角) is also called the **central fibrous body** (中心纤维体), which is located between the mitral annulus, the tricuspid annulus and the fibrous ring of the posterior leaflet of the aortic valve. Compared with that of the right fibrous trigone, the volume of **left fibrous trigone** (左纤维三角) is small. It is located between the fibrous ring of left leaflet of the aortic valve and the mitral annulus. It is an important sign of the mitral valve operation.

2.3.2　Wall of the Heart

The wall of the heart is composed of the endocardium, the myocardium and the epicardium, which corresponds to the three layer structure of the blood vessels, respectively. The myocardium is the main part of the wall of the heart.

2.3.2.1　Endocardium

The endocardium is a smooth membrane that is covered on the intracardiac surface. It is composed of endothelium and subendothelial layer.

2.3.2.2　Myocardium

The myocardium is the main body of the heart wall, including atrial muscles and ventricular muscles. These two types of muscles are separated by the fibrous skeleton. Therefore, the atrium and the ventricles do not contract at the same time.

The atrial muscles are present as grid shape, most-

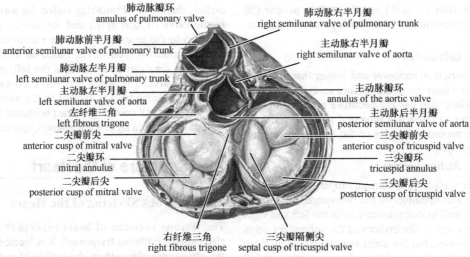

Figure 2-6   Fibrous trigones and annuli (superior view).

ly composed of the pectinate muscles. The atrial muscles are thin and consist of two layers. The muscles of superficial layers surround the left and right atria, and the muscles of deep layer are the proper muscles of the left and right atria.

Compared with the atrial muscles, the ventricular muscles are thicker, especially in the left ventricle. The myocardium can be divided into superficial layer, middle layer, and deep layer. The middle layer is the thickest and surrounds the left and right ventricles, respectively.

2.3.2.3   Epicardium

The epicardium is the visceral layer of the serous pericardium that covers the myocardial surface.

2.3.3   Interatrial and Interventricular Septums

2.3.3.1   Interatrial septum

The interatrial septum is located between the left and right atria, which is formed by the myocardium and connective tissue. On the right side of the interatrial septum, there is an oval fossa, which is the thinnest part of the septum.

2.3.3.2   Interventricular septum

The interventricular septum is located between the left and right ventricles, and it can be divided into a muscular part and a membranous part.

The **muscular part** (肌部) is formed by the myocardium and the endocardium. It takes up most of the interventricular septum, and its thickness is at about 1–2 centimeters. On the left side, there is the left bundle branch under the endocardium, and on right side, there is the right bundle branch.

The **membranous part** (膜部) is located at the junction of the atrium and the ventricle. Its upper boundary is the aortic valve. The anterior boundary is the muscular part of the interventricular septum,

and the posterior boundary is the right atrial wall. The membranous part can be divided into atrioventricular and interventricular parts by the septal leaflet of the tricuspid annulus. The interventricular part is smaller, and the interventricular septal defects usually occur in this region.

2.3.3.3   Atrioventricular septum

It is the transitional and overlapping area between the interatrial septum and the interventricular septum.

2.4   Conduction System of the Heart

The cardiac myocytes can be divided into two types according to morphology and function. They are autorhythmic cells and contractile cells. The contractile cells are the main component of atrial walls and ventricular walls, and their main function is contraction. The autorhythmic cells can generate and transmit electrical impulses. The conduction system of the heart includes the sinoatrial node, the internodal tracts, the atrioventricular node, the atrioventricular bundle, the left and right bundle branches, and the Purkinje fibers.

2.4.1   Sinoatrial Node

The **sinoatrial node** (窦房结) is the normal pacing point of the heart, which is semilunar shaped. It is located deep in the epicardium at the upper 1/3 of the sulcus terminalis. In addition to **pacemaker cells** (起搏细胞) and **transitional cells** (过渡细胞), there are plenty of collagen fibers in the sinoatrial node, forming a reticular scaffold.

2.4.2   Internodal Tracts

The conductive pathway of electrical impulses produced in sinoatrial node is not fully understood so far.

However, there are three internodal tracts connecting the sinoatrial and atrioventricular nodes. The anterior internodal tract arises from the sinoatrial node and divides into the superior internodal tract (Bachmann tract) and the descending branch at the upper margin of the interatrial septum. The superior internodal tract distributes on the anterior wall of left atrium, while the descending branch runs to the upper margin of the atrioventricular node. The middle internodal tract arises from the sinoatrial node. It goes around the superior vena cava and then to the interatrial septum, finally descends anterior to the fossa ovalis. The posterior internodal tract arises from the lower end of the sinoatrial node. It descends within the crista terminalis, and then reaches the posterior margin of the atrioventricular node.

2.4.3　Atrioventricular Node

The **atrioventricular node** (房室结) is the central part of the atrioventricular junction region and is located at the tip of Koch Triangle. The main function of the atrioventricular node is to transmit electrical impulses to the ventricular muscles and to produce ventricular contraction.

2.4.4　Atrioventricular Bundle

The **atrioventricular bundle** (房室束) arises from the anterior part of the atrioventricular node, and is also called **His bundle** (希氏束). It passes through the central fibrous body, running between the muscular part of interventricular septum and the central fibrous body, then traverses the membranous part of interventricular septum, finally divides into the right bundle branch and the left bundle branch.

2.4.5　Left Bundle Branch

The **left bundle branch** (左束支) extends from the atrioventricular bundle and runs under the left endocardium of the interventricular septum. It separates into anterior, septal, and posterior groups at the muscular part of interventricular septum, and finally reaches all parts of the left ventricle.

2.4.6　Right Bundle Branch

The **right bundle branch** (右束支) extends from the atrioventricular bundle and distributes in the anterior papillary muscle and the right ventricular wall.

2.4.7　Purkinje Fibers

The **Purkinje fibers** (浦肯野纤维) are the networks formed by the branches of the left and right bundle branches under the endocardium. They are mainly distributed in the cardiac apex, papillary muscles, and other areas.

2.5　Vessels of the Heart

The circulation of blood within the heart is called the coronary circulation. The blood supply to the heart is from the left and right coronary arteries. Most of the venous blood flows back into the right atrium through the coronary sinus. A part of it flows directly into the right atrium and there are a few more inflows into the left atrium and the left and right ventricles directly.

2.5.1　Coronary Arteries

2.5.1.1　Left coronary artery

The **left coronary artery** (左冠状动脉) (Fig. 2-2) arises from the left aortic sinus. Its trunk is short, about 5–10 millimeters in length. The left coronary artery runs between the left auricle and the pulmonary trunk, and then divides into the **anterior interventricular branch** (前室间支) and the **circumflex branch** (旋支) at the coronary sulcus. The left coronary artery and its branches nourish the left atrium and ventricle, the adjacent part of the right ventricle, and the anterior part of the interventricular septum.

1) Anterior interventricular branch: It can be seen as a direct continuation of the left coronary artery. The anterior interventricular branch runs in the anterior interventricular groove of the cardiac apex, which anastomoses with the posterior interventricular branch on the right side of the apex. The anterior interventricular branch and its branches nourish the left anterior ventricular wall, the anterior papillary muscle, the cardiac apex, the part of right anterior ventricular wall, the anterior 2/3 of the interventricular septum, and the left and right bundle branches of the conduction system.

The branches of the anterior interventricular branch include the left anterior ventricular branch, the right anterior ventricular branch, and the anterior branch of the interventricular septum.

2) Circumflex branch: It is also called left circumflex branch. The circumflex branch runs in the coronary sulcus from the right side to the left side. It goes around the left border of the heart, finally reaches the diaphragmatic surface. The circumflex branch and its branches distribute in the left atrium, the small part of left anterior ventricular wall, the lateral wall of the left ventricle, and the left posterior ventricular wall.

The branches of the circumflex branch include the left marginal branch, the left posterior ventricular branch, the branch of sinoatrial node, the atrial branch, and the left atrial circumflex branch.

2.5.1.2　Right coronary artery

The **right coronary artery** (右冠状动脉) (Fig. 2-2, Fig. 2-3) arises from the right aortic sinus. It runs in the coronary sulcus from the left side to the right side, between the right auricle and the pulmonary trunk, and finally reaches the coronary sulcus on the diaphragmatic surface. The right coronary artery usually divides into the **posterior interventricular branch** (后室间支) and the **right circumflex branch** (右旋支) near the atrioventricular crux.

In addition to the posterior interventricular branch and the right circumflex branch, the branches of the right coronary artery also include the branch of sinoatrial node, the right marginal branch, the right atrial branch, and the branch of atrioventricular node.

The right coronary artery and its branches distribute in the right atrium, the most part of the right anterior ventricular wall, the lateral wall of the right ventricle, the posterior wall of the right ventricle, the part of the left posterior ventricular wall, the posterior 1/3 of interventricular septum, the sinoatrial node, the atrioventricular node, and the left bundle branch.

2.5.2 Cardiac Veins

The veins of the heart can be divided into two systems: the superficial veins and the deep veins. The superficial veins arise from the myocardium. They converge into the network or trunk under the epicardium, and finally get collected by the coronary sinus and flow into the right atrium. The deep veins also arise from the myocardium, which directly converge into the chamber of the heart, especially the right atrium (Fig. 2-2, Fig. 2-3).

2.5.2.1 Coronary sinus

The **coronary sinus** (冠状窦) is located in the coronary sulcus on the diaphragmatic surface of the heart, between the left atrium and left ventricle. It opens into the right atrium through the orifice of the coronary sinus, which drains the large majority of the venous blood from the heart. The tributaries of the coronary sinus include the great cardiac vein, the middle cardiac vein and the small cardiac vein.

1) Great cardiac vein (心大静脉): It runs along with the anterior interventricular branch of the left coronary artery in the anterior interventricular groove, and then enters the coronary sinus through the coronary sulcus.

2) Middle cardiac vein (心中静脉): It arises from the cardiac apex. The middle cardiac vein ascends in the posterior interventricular groove, and finally enters the coronary sinus. In the course, it runs along with the posterior interventricular branch of the right coronary artery.

3) Small cardiac vein (心小静脉): It runs in the coronary sulcus along with the right coronary artery, and finally enters either the coronary sinus or the middle cardiac vein.

2.5.2.2 Anterior cardiac vein

There are approximately 1–4 anterior cardiac veins arising from the right anterior ventricular wall. They directly enter the right atrium, and some of the **anterior cardiac veins** (心前静脉) anastomose with the smallest cardiac vein.

2.5.2.3 Smallest cardiac vein

The **smallest cardiac vein** (心最小静脉) is also called the Thebesius vein. They are the small veins in the cardiac wall, which open directly into the cardiac cavities.

2.6 Pericardium

The **pericardium** (心包) (Fig. 2-7) is the conical fibrous serous capsule that encloses the heart and the roots of the great vessels. It has two layers. The outer layer is the fibrous pericardium, and the inner layer is the serous pericardium.

2.6.1 Fibrous Pericardium

The **fibrous pericardium** (纤维心包) is made up of tough fibrous connective tissues. In the upper aspect, it is continuous with the adventitia of the great vessels, like ascending aorta, pulmonary trunk, and so

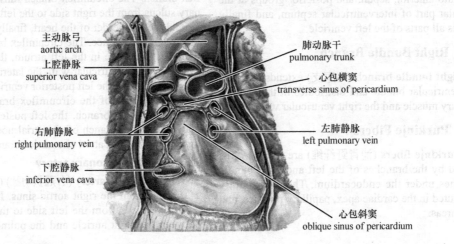

主动脉弓 aortic arch
上腔静脉 superior vena cava
右肺静脉 right pulmonary vein
下腔静脉 inferior vena cava
肺动脉干 pulmonary trunk
心包横窦 transverse sinus of pericardium
左肺静脉 left pulmonary vein
心包斜窦 oblique sinus of pericardium

Figure 2-7 Pericardium.

on. In the lower aspects, it attaches to the central tendon of the diaphragm.

2.6.2　Serous Pericardium

The **serous pericardium** (浆膜心包) can be divided into the visceral layer and parietal layer. The parietal layer is in close contact with the fibrous pericardium while the visceral layer covers the outermost surface of the myocardium, forming the epicardium. Between the two layers, there is a closed space called **pericardial cavity** (心包腔).

The recesses of the pericardial cavity are called **pericardial sinuses** (心包窦). They are the **transverse sinus of pericardium** (心包横窦), the **oblique sinus of pericardium** (心包斜窦), and the **anteroinferior sinus of pericardium** (心包前下窦).

Summary

心脏是一个中空的肌性纤维性器官，斜位于胸腔的中纵隔内，外裹心包。可分为一尖、一底、两面、三缘（心尖、心底、胸肋面、膈面、下缘、左缘和右缘），其表面有冠状沟、前室间沟、后室间沟和后房间沟，可作为心腔的表面分界。心被心间隔分为左、右心房和左、右心室，同侧心房和心室借房室口相通。心纤维支架位于房室口、肺动脉口和主动脉口的周围，致密的结缔组织，包括左右纤维三角，四个瓣纤维环（肺动脉瓣环、主动脉瓣环、二尖瓣环和三尖瓣环），圆锥韧带，室间隔膜部和瓣膜间隔等。

心传导系是由特殊心肌细胞构成，包括窦房结、结间束、房室交界区、房室束、左、右束支和Purkinje（浦肯野）纤维。供应心脏的血液来自左、右冠状动脉，而心回流的静脉血，绝大部分经冠状窦汇入右心房。

学生在学习心血管系统的解剖学知识过程中，应重点学习心脏的位置、外形，尤其是四个心腔内的特殊结构，如卵圆窝、冠状窦口、三尖瓣复合体、二尖瓣复合体等。此外，心传导系也是心脏解剖学知识的重点。对于心的血管、心包和体表投影，学生应达到熟练掌握的程度。

Zhang Shanqiang, Wang Lulu (张善强, 王璐璐)

Chapter 3   Artery

Any blood vessel that carries blood away from the heart can be called an artery. In human body, the distribution of arteries is different. For example, the distribution of arteries in the head, neck, pelvis and limbs is symmetrical, while the distribution of arteries in the thoracic and abdominal cavities is asymmetrical. The aorta arises from the left ventricle and its branches carry arterial blood, while the pulmonary trunk arises from the right ventricle and its branches transport venous blood. The segment of the artery before it enters an organ is called the external organ artery, and the segment of the artery within the organ is called the internal organ artery.

3.1   Arteries of Pulmonary Circulation

The pulmonary trunk, located in the pericardium, is a stubby artery, arises from the right ventricle and divides into the left and right pulmonary arteries beneath the aortic arch. The **left pulmonary artery** (左肺动脉) is short. It transversely runs in front of the left main bronchus, and divides into superior and inferior branches before they enter the upper and lower pulmonary lobes. The **right pulmonary artery** (右肺动脉) is longer and thicker. Behind the ascending aorta and superior vena cava, it transversely runs to the right side, and divides into the superior, middle, and inferior branches before they enter the three lobes of the right lung. The **arterial ligament** (动脉韧带) is a fibrous connective tissue cord between the bifurcation of the pulmonary trunk and the lower edge of the aortic arch.

3.2   Arteries of Systemic Circulation

3.2.1   Aorta

The **aorta** (主动脉) of the systemic circulation arises from the left ventricle, and its full length can be divided into three segments. The **ascending aorta** (升主动脉) is the first segment, which is located between the upper margin of the left ventricle and the second ster-nocostal joint. The second segment is the **aortic arch** (主动脉弓), located between the second sternocostal joint to the lower edge of the fourth thoracic vertebra.

From right to left side, the three branches of the aortic arch are the **brachiocephalic trunk** (头臂干), the **left common carotid artery** (左颈总动脉), and the **left subclavian artery** (左锁骨下动脉). The brachiocephalic trunk can be further divided into the **right common carotid artery** (右颈总动脉) and the **right subclavian artery** (右锁骨下动脉) at the level of the right sternoclavicular joint. Under the adventitia of the aortic arch, the rich nerve endings that can feel the change of blood pressure are called pressure receptors. Beneath the aortic arch, the 2–3 millet like structures near the arterial ligament are called the **aortic glomera** (主动脉小球). These structures are chemical receptors, which can feel the changes in the partial pressure of carbon dioxide, partial pressure of oxygen and hydrogen ion concentration in the blood. The third segment which is located between the lower edge of the fourth thoracic vertebra and the lower edge of the fourth lumbar vertebra, is called the **descending aorta** (降主动脉). It can be divided into the **thoracic aorta** (胸主动脉) and the **abdominal aorta** (腹主动脉) by the aortic hiatus at the level of twelfth thoracic vertebra. Finally, the descending aorta divides into the left and right **common iliac arteries** (髂总动脉) at the lower edge of the fourth lumbar vertebra.

3.2.2   Arteries of Head and Neck

The **common carotid artery** (颈总动脉) (Fig. 3-1, Fig. 3-2) is the main arterial trunk of the head and neck. The left common carotid artery arises from the aortic arch, while the right common carotid artery arises from the brachiocephalic trunk. Both the arteries ascend along the lateral sides of the trachea and esophagus through the posterior aspect of the sternoclavicular articulation. Finally, the two common carotid arteries divide into the **external carotid artery** (颈外动脉) and **internal cartoid artery** (颈内动脉) at the level of the upper border of the thyroid cartilage. The position of the upper segment of the common carotid artery is superficial, and the pulsation of the artery can be felt on the living body. Near the bifurcation of the common carotid artery, there are **carotid sinus** (颈动脉窦) and **carotid glomus** (颈动脉小球).

Near the ending of the common carotid artery and the beginning of the internal carotid artery, there is a slight dilation called carotid sinus which contains rich

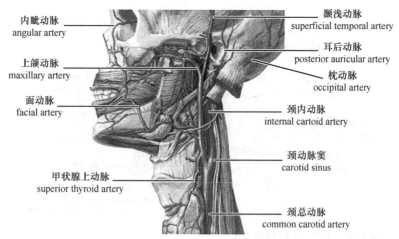

内眦动脉 angular artery		颞浅动脉 superficial temporal artery
上颌动脉 maxillary artery		耳后动脉 posterior auricular artery
面动脉 facial artery		枕动脉 occipital artery
		颈内动脉 internal cartoid artery
		颈动脉窦 carotid sinus
甲状腺上动脉 superior thyroid artery		颈总动脉 common carotid artery

Figure 3-1　The arteries of the head and neck.

supply of nerve endings and can play the function of the pressure receptor regulating the blood pressure.

The carotid glomus is also called carotid body. It is an elliptical structure which connects the posterior surface of the bifurcation of the common carotid artery by connective tissues. It is the chemical receptor which can feel the changes in the partial pressure of carbon dioxide, partial pressure of oxygen and hydrogen ion concentration in the blood.

3.2.2.1　External carotid artery

Firstly, the external carotid artery is located at the anteromedial side of the internal carotid artery. During its ascent, the external carotid artery moves to the lateral side of the internal carotid artery.

The branches of the external carotid artery include the **superior thyroid artery** (甲状腺上动脉), the **lingual artery** (舌动脉), the **facial artery** (面动脉), the **superficial temporal artery** (颞浅动脉), the **maxillary artery** (上颌动脉), the **occipital artery** (枕动脉), the **posterior auricular artery** (耳后动脉), and the **ascending pharyngeal artery** (咽升动脉).

The superficial temporal artery and the maxillary artery are the two terminal branches of the external carotid artery. The important branch of the maxillary artery is the **middle meningeal artery** (脑膜中动脉), that has the anterior and posterior branches, and the anterior branch runs at the internal surface of the pterion.

3.2.2.2　Internal carotid artery

The internal carotid artery (Fig. 3-1) has no branches around the neck. Soon after it originates from the common carotid artery, it ascends to the skull base, and enters the cranial cavity through the carotid canal. The branches of the internal carotid artery are distributed to the visual organs and the brain.

3.2.2.3　Subclavian artery

The origins of the two subclavian arteries are differ-ent. The left subclavian artery arises from the aortic arch, while the right subclavian artery arises from the brachiocephalic trunk. During their course, both of the two arteries obliquely enter the roots of the neck through the posterior aspect of the sternoclavicular articulation. They form a curve in front of the cupula of pleura, pass through the scalene fissure, and cross-es over the outer edge of the first rib to become the axillary artery.

The branches of the subclavian artery include the **vertebral artery** (椎动脉), the **internal thoracic artery** (胸廓内动脉), the **thyrocervical trunk** (甲状颈干), and the **costocervical trunk** (肋颈干) (Fig. 3-2).

The vertebral artery arises from the subclavian artery at the medial side of the scalenus anterior, and runs superiorly through the transverse foramina of the upper six cervical vertebrae, and enters the cranial cavity through the foramen magnum. The branches of the vertebral artery are distributed in the brain and spinal cord.

The internal thoracic artery arises from the sub-clavian artery, at about the opposite side of the origin of the vertebral artery. It descends into the thoracic cavity, and its branches are distributed in the anterior thoracic wall, the pericardium, diaphragm, and the breast.

The thyrocervical trunk is a short trunk located at the medial side of the scalenus anterior. It arises from the lateral side of the subclavian artery, and then divides into the inferior thyroid artery, the suprascap-ular artery, and other branches.

At the lateral side of the thyrocervical trunk, the costocervical trunk (Fig. 3-2) arises from the subcla-vian artery. It is also a short trunk, which divides into some branches and is distributed in the deep cervical muscles and the posterior part of the first and second intercostal space.

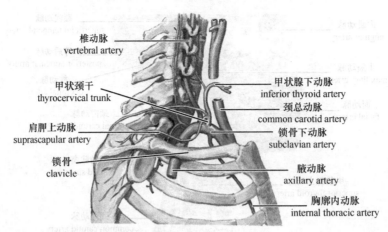

Figure 3-2 The subclavian artery and its branches.

3.2.3 Arteries of Upper Limb

3.2.3.1 Axillary artery

The **axillary artery** (腋动脉) (Fig. 3-3) is the direct continuation of the subclavian artery at the outer edge of the first rib. It descends through the deep part of the axilla and becomes the brachial artery at the lower border of the latissimus dorsi. The branches of axillary artery include the **superior thoracic** artery (胸上动脉), the **thoracoacromial artery** (胸肩峰动脉), the **lateral thoracic artery** (胸外侧动脉), the **subscapular artery** (肩胛下动脉), the **anterior circumflex humeral artery** (旋肱前动脉), and the **posterior circumflex humeral artery** (旋肱后动脉).

The superior thoracic artery is distributed in the first and second intercostal space.

The thoracoacromial artery and its branches supply the pectoralis major, pectoralis minor, deltoid and shoulder joint.

The lateral thoracic artery is accompanied by the long thoracic nerve, which is distributed in the serratus anterior, the pectoralis major, the pectoralis minor and the breast.

The subscapular artery can be divided into the tho-

racodorsal artery and the circumflex scapular artery. The thoracodorsal artery is distributed in the latissimus dorsi and the serratus anterior. The circumflex scapular artery reaches the infraspinous fossa through the triangular foramen, and then anastomoses with the suprascapular artery.

The anterior circumflex humeral artery nourishes the shoulder joint and the adjacent muscles.

The posterior circumflex humeral artery is accompanied by the axillary nerve. After they pass through the quadrilateral foramen, the artery wraps around the surgical neck of the humerus to nourish the deltoid and the shoulder joint.

3.2.3.2 Brachial artery

The **brachial artery** (肱动脉) is the direct continuation of the axillary artery. It runs together with the median nerve in the medial sulcus of the biceps brachii and divides into the **radial artery** (桡动脉) and **ulnar artery** (尺动脉) at the level of the radial neck. The position of the brachial artery is superficial and its pulsation can be palpated at the medial sulcus of the biceps brachii. The important branch of the brachial artery is the **deep brachial artery** (肱深动脉), it is accompanied by the radial nerve along the sulcus

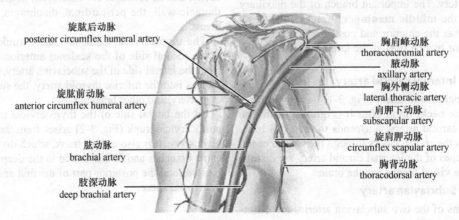

Figure 3-3 The axillary artery.

of the radial nerve, and its branches nourish the triceps brachii and humerus. The terminal branches of the deep brachial artery participate in the composition of the arterial network of the elbow joint. The other branches of the brachial artery also include the **superior ulnar collateral artery** (尺侧上副动脉), the **inferior ulnar collateral artery** (尺侧下副动脉), and so on.

The radial artery runs between the brachioradialis and the pronator teres at first, and then descends between the tendons of the brachioradialis and the flexor carpi radialis. It reaches the dorsum of the hand by wrapping around the styloid process of the radius, and finally reaches the palm through the first metacarpal space. The end of the radial artery anastomoses with the deep palmar branch of the ulnar artery to form the **deep palmar arch** (掌深弓). The main branches of the radial artery include the **superficial palmar branch** (掌浅支) and the **principal artery of thumb** (拇主要动脉). The superficial palmar branch anastomoses with the ulnar artery to form the **superficial palmar arch** (掌浅弓).

The ulnar artery descends between the flexor carpi ulnaris and the flexor digitorum superficialis, and then along the radial side of the pisiform bone to reach the palm. The branches of the ulnar artery nourish the muscles of the ulnar side of the forearm and participate in the composition of the arterial network of the elbow joint. The main branches of the ulnar artery include the **common interosseous artery** (骨间总动脉) and the **deep palmar branch** (掌深支). The common interosseous artery can be divided into the **anterior interosseous artery** (骨间前动脉) and **posterior interosseous artery** (骨间后动脉). They descend along the anterior and posterior surfaces of the interosseous membrane of the forearm, respectively. The two arteries and their branches nourish the muscles of the forearm, ulna and radius.

The superficial palmar arch (Fig. 3-4) is formed by the ends of the ulnar artery and the branch of superficial palmar artery, which is located in the deep region of the palmar aponeurosis. It has four branches, which include three **common palmar digital arteries** (指掌侧总动脉) and one **ulnar palmar artery of little finger** (小指尺侧动脉). Each common palmar digital artery can be divided into two **proper palmar digital arteries** (指掌侧固有动脉) near the metacarpophalangeal joint and is distributed in the relative margin of fingers 2 to 5. The ulnar palmar artery of quinary finger is distributed in the ulnar margin of the palmar surface of the little finger.

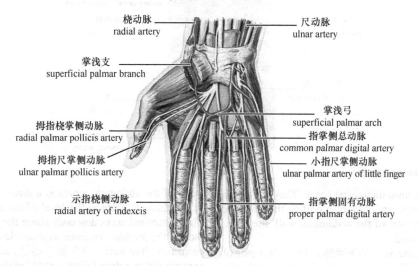

Figure 3-4   The superficial palmar arch.

The deep palmar arch (Fig. 3-5) is formed by the ends of the radial artery and the deep palmar branch of the ulnar artery, which is located in the deep region of the flexor digitorum profundus. The branches of the arch include the three **palmar metacarpal arteries** (掌心动脉), and the three arteries join together to form the three common palmar digital arteries, respectively.

3.2.4   Arteries of Thorax

The thoracic aorta (Fig. 3-6) is the arterial trunk of the thorax, which is located in the posterior mediastinum of the thoracic cavity. It is the continuation of the aortic arch at the left side of the fourth thoracic vertebra. It descends along the left side of the spinal cord, and passes through the aortic hiatus to become the abdominal aorta at the level of the twelfth thoracic vertebra. The branches of the thoracic aorta include the parietal and visceral branches.

3.2.4.1   Parietal branches

1) Posterior intercostal arteries (肋间后动脉): There are 9 pairs of these arteries, which are distrib-

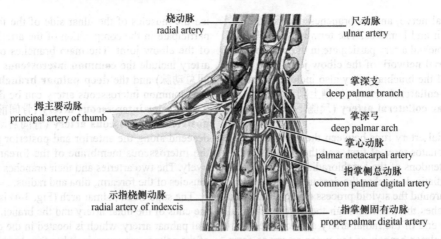

桡动脉
radial artery

尺动脉
ulnar artery

掌深支
deep palmar branch

掌深弓
deep palmar arch

拇主要动脉
principal artery of thumb

掌心动脉
palmar metacarpal artery

指掌侧总动脉
common palmar digital artery

示指桡侧动脉
radial artery of indexcis

指掌侧固有动脉
proper palmar digital artery

Figure 3-5 The deep palmar arch.

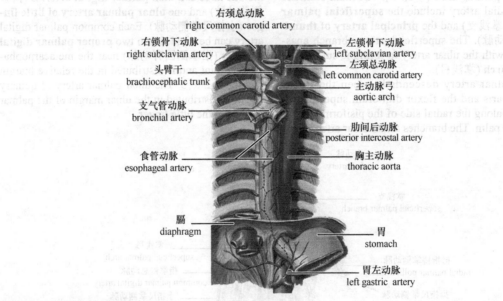

右颈总动脉
right common carotid artery

右锁骨下动脉
right subclavian artery

头臂干
brachiocephalic trunk

支气管动脉
bronchial artery

食管动脉
esophageal artery

膈
diaphragm

左锁骨下动脉
left subclavian artery

左颈总动脉
left common carotid artery

主动脉弓
aortic arch

肋间后动脉
posterior intercostal artery

胸主动脉
thoracic aorta

胃
stomach

胃左动脉
left gastric artery

Figure 3-6 Thoracic aorta.

uted below the third intercostal space. They run along the costal groove and supply blood to the thoracic wall, the upper part of the abdominal wall, the back, and the spinal cord.

2) Subcostal arteries (肋下动脉): There is a pair of these arteries, which are located below the twelfth rib. They supply blood to the corresponding area.

3) Superior phrenic arteries (膈上动脉): There is a pair of these arteries, which supply blood to the posterior part of the diaphragm.

3.2.4.2 Visceral branches

The visceral branches of the thoracic aorta are very small. They include the **bronchial arteries (支气管动脉)**, the **esophageal arteries (食管动脉)**, the pericardial arteries, and so on.

3.2.5 Arteries of Abdomen

The abdominal aorta (Fig. 3-7) is the main arterial

trunk of the abdomen, which is a direct continuation of the thoracic aorta at the level of the aortic hiatus. The abdominal aorta descends along the anterior surface of the lumbar vertebrae, and divides into the **left common iliac artery (左髂总动脉)** and the **right common iliac artery (右髂总动脉)** at the level of the lower edge of the fourth lumbar vertebra. The abdominal aorta also has the parietal branches and visceral branches.

3.2.5.1 Parietal branches

1) Inferior phrenic arteries (膈下动脉): There is a pair of these arteries, which are distributed in the diaphragm and abdominal wall. The superior suprarenal arteries arising from these arteries supply blood to the adrenal gland.

2) Lumbar arteries (腰动脉): The four pairs of lumbar arteries are distributed in the waist, the abdominal wall, and the spinal cord.

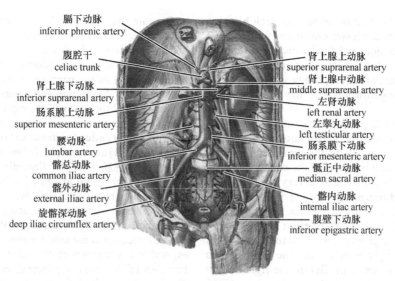

Figure 3-7 Abdominal aorta.

3) Median sacral artery (骶正中动脉): The median sacral artery arises from the posterior part of the bifurcation of the abdominal aorta, which nourishes the sacrum and its surrounding structure.

3.2.5.2 Visceral branches

The visceral branches can be divided into two types: paired and unpaired.

1) Paired branches: The paired branches include the **middle suprarenal arteries** (肾上腺中动脉), the **renal arteries** (肾动脉), the **testicular arteries** (睾丸动脉) (in male) or the **ovarian arteries** (卵巢动脉) (in female).

The middle suprarenal arteries arise from the lateral sides of the abdominal aorta at the level of the first lumbar vertebra. They anastomose with the superior suprarenal arteries and inferior suprarenal arteries in the adrenal gland.

The renal arteries arise from the abdominal aorta at the level of the 1–2 lumbar intervertebral disc. Before they enter the kidney, the renal arteries give off the inferior suprarenal arteries.

Under the point of origin of the renal arteries, the testicular arteries arise from the anterior wall of the abdominal aorta. They are long and small, which descend along the psoas major and enter the scrotum through inguinal canal. In the scrotum, the testicular arteries become the internal spermatic arteries, which are distributed around the testis and epididymis. In females, the corresponding arteries are called the ovarian arteries. They enter the pelvic cavity through the suspensory ligament of ovary, and are distributed around the ovaries and fallopian tubes.

2) Unpaired branches: They are the **celiac trunk** (腹腔干), the **superior mesenteric artery** (肠系膜上动脉), and the **inferior mesenteric artery** (肠系膜下动脉).

The celiac trunk (Fig. 3-8) is a thick and short arterial trunk located beneath the aortic hiatus, and it arises from the anterior wall of the abdominal aorta, and then divides into the **left gastric artery** (胃左动脉), the **common hepatic artery** (肝总动脉), and the **splenic artery** (脾动脉).

The left gastric artery runs towards the upper left direction and reaches the cardia of stomach. It runs

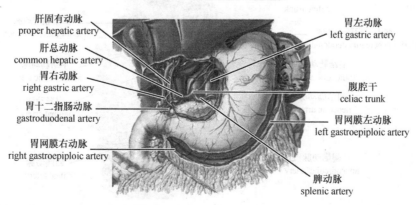

Figure 3-8 The celiac trunk and its branches.

along the lesser curvature of the stomach between the two layers of the lesser omentum, from the left side to the right side, and finally anastomoses with the right gastric artery. Its branches are distributed in the abdominal part of the esophagus, the cardia of the stomach, and the gastric wall near the lesser curvature of the stomach.

The common hepatic artery runs to the right side, and then enters the hepatoduodenal ligament through the upper margin of the superior part of the duodenum. The two branches of the common hepatic artery are the **proper hepatic artery** (肝固有动脉) and the **gastroduodenal artery** (胃十二指肠动脉). The proper hepatic artery runs in the hepatoduodenal ligament, and then gives off the **right gastric artery** (胃右动脉). The proper hepatic artery also gives off the left and right branches, and the two branches are distributed in the liver. Before the right branch enters the liver, it gives off the **cystic artery** (胆囊动脉), which is distributed in the gallbladder. The gastroduodenal artery reaches the lower border of the stomach through the superior part of duodenum and the posterior part of the pylorus of the stomach, and then divides into the **right gastroepiploic artery** (胃网膜右动脉) and the **superior pancreaticoduodenal artery** (胰十二指肠上动脉). The right gastroepiploic artery is distributed around the greater curvature and the greater omentum of the stomach, and its terminal branches anastomose with the left gastroepiploic artery. The superior pancreaticoduodenal artery gives off the anterior and posterior branches, which are distributed around the head of the pancreas and the duodenum.

The splenic artery runs along the upper border of the pancreas to the left side and gives off the branches before it enters the spleen. The branches include the **posterior gastric arteries** (胃后动脉), the **pancreatic branches** (胰支), the **short gastric arteries** (胃短动脉), the **left gastroepiploic artery** (胃网膜左动脉), and the **splenic branches** (脾支).

Beneath the celiac trunk, the superior mesenteric artery (Fig. 3-9) arises from the anterior wall of the abdominal aorta at the level of the first lumbar vertebra. It descends to the posterior aspect through the head and body of the pancreas, crosses the horizontal part of the duodenum, and enters the root of the mesentery, and then runs to the right iliac fossa. The branches of the superior mesenteric artery include the **inferior pancreaticoduodenal artery** (胰十二指肠下动脉), the **jejunal arteries** (空肠动脉) and the **ileal arteries** (回肠动脉), the **ileocolic artery** (回结肠动脉), the **right colic artery** (右结肠动脉), and the **middle colic artery** (中结肠动脉).

The inferior pancreaticoduodenal artery runs between the head of the pancreas and the duodenum. It can be divided into the anterior and posterior branches, and anastomoses with the anterior and posterior branches of the superior pancreaticoduodenal artery. The branches of the inferior pancreaticoduodenal artery supply blood to the pancreas and the duodenum.

The jejunal arteries and the ileal arteries arise from the left wall of the superior mesenteric artery. There are a total of about 13–18 arteries, which run through the mesentery. The jejunal arteries and the ileal arteries give off the branches and anastomose with each other to form the multistage arterial arches. The last stage arch directly enters the small intestine and is distributed in the jejunum and ileum.

The ileocolic artery arises from the right wall of the superior mesenteric artery. The ileocolic artery and its branches supply blood to the terminal part of the ileum, the cecum, the appendix and ascending colon. The branch of ileocolic artery around the appendix is called **appendicular artery** (阑尾动脉).

The right colic artery and its branches are distributed in the ascending colon, while the middle colic artery and its branches are distributed in the transverse colon.

The inferior mesenteric artery (Fig. 3-10) arises from the anterior wall of the abdominal aorta at the

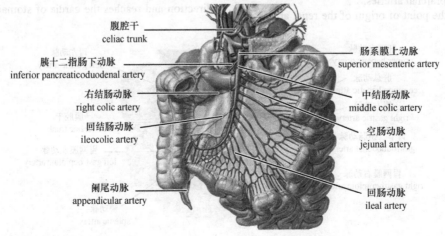

腹腔干
celiac trunk

胰十二指肠下动脉
inferior pancreaticoduodenal artery

右结肠动脉
right colic artery

回结肠动脉
ileocolic artery

阑尾动脉
appendicular artery

肠系膜上动脉
superior mesenteric artery

中结肠动脉
middle colic artery

空肠动脉
jejunal artery

回肠动脉
ileal artery

Figure 3-9　The superior mesenteric artery.

level of the third lumbar vertebra. It runs towards the lower left side and is distributed around the descending colon, the sigmoid colon, and the upper part of the rectum. The branches of the inferior mesenteric artery include the **left colic artery** (左结肠动脉), the **sigmoid arteries** (乙状结肠动脉), and the **superior rectal artery** (直肠上动脉).

The left colic artery and its branches are distributed around the descending colon. The 2–3 sigmoid arteries run towards the lower left side, and their branches anastomose with the left colic artery and the superior rectal artery. The superior rectal artery is the direct continuation of the inferior mesenteric artery, which can be divided into two branches at the level of the third sacral vertebra. The two branches of the superior rectal artery are distributed around the two lateral sides of the upper part of rectum.

3.2.6 Arteries of Pelvis

The left and right common iliac arteries descend along the medial side of the psoas major. Each of them can be divided into the **internal iliac artery** (髂内动脉) and **external iliac artery** (髂外动脉) at the point of the sacroiliac joint (Fig. 3-11).

The internal iliac artery is a short arterial trunk of the pelvis. It descends along the lateral wall of the pelvic cavity, which nourishes the organs and muscles of the pelvis. The branches of the internal iliac artery include the parietal branches and visceral branches.

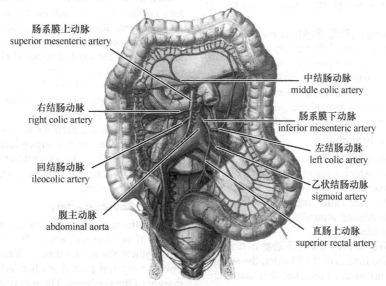

肠系膜上动脉
superior mesenteric artery

中结肠动脉
middle colic artery

右结肠动脉
right colic artery

肠系膜下动脉
inferior mesenteric artery

左结肠动脉
left colic artery

回结肠动脉
ileocolic artery

乙状结肠动脉
sigmoid artery

腹主动脉
abdominal aorta

直肠上动脉
superior rectal artery

Figure 3-10　The inferior mesenteric artery.

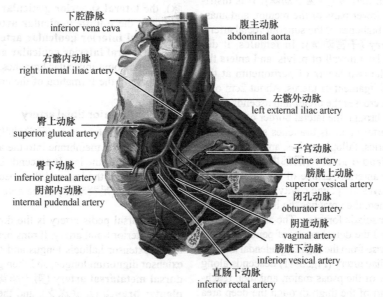

下腔静脉
inferior vena cava

腹主动脉
abdominal aorta

右髂内动脉
right internal iliac artery

左髂外动脉
left external iliac artery

臀上动脉
superior gluteal artery

子宫动脉
uterine artery

臀下动脉
inferior gluteal artery

膀胱上动脉
superior vesical artery

阴部内动脉
internal pudendal artery

闭孔动脉
obturator artery

阴道动脉
vaginal artery

膀胱下动脉
inferior vesical artery

直肠下动脉
inferior rectal artery

Figure 3-11　The arteries of pelvis (in female).

3.2.6.1　Parietal branches

1) Obturator artery (闭孔动脉): It descends along the lateral wall of the pelvis to the anteroinferior side, and then reaches the medial side of the thigh through the obturator membrane. The obturator artery and its branches supply blood to the medial muscular group of the thigh and the hip joint.

2) Superior gluteal artery (臀上动脉): It reaches the buttocks through the suprapiriform foramen. The superior gluteal artery and its branches supply blood to the upper part of the gluteal muscles and the hip joint.

3) Inferior gluteal artery (臀下动脉): It reaches the buttocks through the theinfrapiriform foramen. The inferior gluteal artery and its branches supply blood to the lower part of the gluteal muscles and the hip joint.

4) Iliolumbar artery (髂腰动脉): It arises from the proximal end of the internal iliac artery and is distributed around the iliacus and psoas major.

5) Lateral sacral artery (骶外侧动脉): It descends along the anterior surface of the lateral edge of sacrum and is distributed around the posterior wall of the pelvic cavity and the structures of the sacral canal.

3.2.6.2　Visceral branches

1) Umbilical artery (脐动脉): It is the arterial trunk of the fetal period, which anastomoses with the initial part of the internal iliac artery. The 2–3 branches of the umbilical artery are called superior vesical arteries, which are distributed around the upper and middle part of the bladder.

2) Inferior vesical artery (膀胱下动脉): It is distributed around the fundus of the bladder, the seminal vesicle, and the prostate. In females, it is distributed around the bladder and vagina.

3) Inferior rectal artery (直肠下动脉): It is distributed around the lower parts of the rectum, and anastomoses with the branches of the superior rectal artery.

4) Uterine artery (子宫动脉): In females, it descends along the lateral wall of pelvis, and enters the space between the two layers of peritoneum at the base of the broad ligament of uterus. About 2cm outside the cervix, it crosses the ureter and ascends to the fundus of uterus through the lateral border of the uterus. The uterine artery and its branches supply blood to the uterus, ovaries, fallopian tubes, and vagina.

5) Internal pudendal artery (阴部内动脉): It descends along the anterior surface of the inferior gluteal artery and leaves the pelvic cavity through the infrapiriform foramen, then reaches the ischioanal fossa through the lesser sciatic foramen. The anal artery, the perineal artery, and the dorsal artery of penis or dorsal artery of clitoris arise from the internal pudendal artery.

The external iliac artery (Fig. 3-11) descends along the medial border of the psoas major, and then reaches the anterior part of the thigh through the deep area of the middle point of the inguinal ligament. The femoral artery is the direct continuation of the external iliac artery, and the **inferior epigastric artery** (腹壁下动脉) and **deep iliac circumflex artery** (旋髂深动脉) are branches of the external iliac artery.

3.2.7　Arteries of Lower Limbs

3.2.7.1　Femoral artery

The **femoral artery** (股动脉) is the arterial trunk of the lower limb, which descends through the femoral triangle, and enters the popliteal fossa through the adductor canal to become the popliteal artery. Beneath of the midpoint of the inguinal ligament, the position of the femoral artery is superficial, and the pulsation of the artery can be felt on the living body. The main branch of the femoral artery is the **deep femoral artery** (股深动脉). Beneath the midpoint of the inguinal ligament, about 2–5cm, the deep femoral artery arises from the femoral artery. The deep femoral artery gives off the **medial femoral circumflex artery** (旋股内侧动脉), the **lateral femoral circumflex artery** (旋股外侧动脉), and 3–4 **perforating arteries** (穿动脉) to supply blood to the femur and muscular groups of the thigh.

In addition to the deep femoral artery, the femoral artery also gives off the **superficial epigastric artery** (腹壁浅动脉), the **superficial circumflex iliac artery** (旋髂浅动脉), and the **external pudendal artery** (阴部外动脉).

3.2.7.2　Popliteal artery

The **popliteal artery** (腘动脉) is the direct continuation of the femoral artery. It descends deep into the popliteal fossa, and then divides into the anterior tibial artery and posterior tibial artery at the lower margin of the popliteus. The popliteal artery gives off the **medial superior genicular artery** (膝上内侧动脉), the **lateral superior genicular artery** (膝上外侧动脉), the **middle genicular artery** (膝中动脉), the **medial inferior genicular artery** (膝下内侧动脉), the **lateral inferior genicular artery** (膝下外侧动脉), and some muscular branches. These branches participate in the formation of the arterial network of the knee joint.

3.2.7.3　Anterior tibial artery

The **anterior tibial artery** (胫前动脉) pierces through the interosseous membrane into the anterior muscular compartment of the leg. It descends between the anterior muscles of the leg, and then becomes the **dorsal pedis artery** (足背动脉) at the anterior aspect of the ankle joint.

The dorsal pedis artery is the direct continuation of the anterior tibial artery. It runs between the tendon of the extensor hallucis longus and the tendon of the extensor digitorum longus, and then gives off the **first dorsal metatarsal artery** (第一跖背动脉), the **deep plantar branch** (足底深支), and the **arcuate artery** (弓状动脉) at the proximal side of the first metatarsal space.

3.2.7.4　Posterior tibial artery

In the posterior part of the leg, the **posterior tibial artery** (胫后动脉) descends between the superficial muscles and deep muscles. It reaches the plantar through the posterior side of the medial ankle, and finally divides into the medial and lateral plantar arteries. In addition to the two branches, the peroneal artery is an important branch of the posterior tibial artery.

1) Peroneal artery (腓动脉): It arises from the upper part of the posterior tibial artery, which descends along the medial side of the fibula. The peroneal artery and its branches nourish the adjacent muscles, the tibia, and the fibula.

2) Medial plantar artery (足底内侧动脉): It runs along the medial side of the sole, which distributes around the medial side of the pelma.

3) Lateral plantar artery (足底外侧动脉): It runs from the lateral side of the pelma to the fifth metatarsal bone, and then turns to the left side to reach the first metatarsal space. The lateral plantar artery anastomoses with the deep plantar branch to form the plantar arch, and the plantar arch gives off branches to distribute around the toes.

Summary

动脉是输送血液离开心脏到全身各器官的血管。由左心室发出的主动脉及各级分支运送动脉血至全身各处（肺除外）毛细血管进行物质交换；而由右心室发出的肺动脉干及其分支则输送静脉血至肺进行气体交换。

这一部分知识中，学生除掌握肺循环和体循环的基本知识外，还要沿着体循环的动脉主干（主动脉）进行分段学习：升主动脉——发出的左、右冠状动脉；主动脉弓——与升主动脉以胸骨角平面为界，向左分出的头臂干、左颈总动脉和左锁骨下动脉；降主动脉——与主动脉的分界标志是第4胸椎体下缘，以膈为界分为上段的胸主动脉和下段的腹主动脉。

在熟记全身各部主要动脉及其分支后，运用画图法或图表法会对加强记忆与理解具有良好的帮助。

Zhang Shanqiang, Wang Lulu (张善强, 王璐璐)

Chapter 4   Vein

The veins are the blood vessels that carry the blood back to the heart, which originate from the capillaries and end in the atrium. The number of veins is more than that of the arteries, the diameter of the vein is thicker and the lumen is larger. Compared with the accompanying artery, the wall of the vein is thin and soft, and the elasticity is small. The veins of the specimen collapse and contain blood stasis. In terms of structure and distribution, the veins have the following characteristics.

In human body, the veins usually have semilunar-shaped venous valve. The valves are usually paired, with the free margin of the valve is usually oriented towards the heart. The main function of the venous valve is to prevent the reflux of the blood. In the vein of the human body, the veins of the extremities have more venous valves, while the veins in the trunk have little venous or no venous valves.

The veins of systemic circulation can be divided into two kinds: the **superficial veins** (浅静脉) and the **deep veins** (深静脉). The superficial veins are located in the superficial subcutaneous fascia, also known as the subcutaneous veins. The superficial veins do not accompany the arteries, and finally join into the deep veins. The deep veins are located in the deep fascia, they accompany the arteries and are also known as the **accompanying veins** (伴行静脉). The name and course of the deep veins are same with the accompanying arteries, and the drainage range and distribution are also same.

The venous anastomosis is rich. The superficial veins anastomose with each other in the hands and feet to form the venous network, while the deep veins form the venous plexus around the organs. There are abundant traffic branches between the superficial veins, the deep veins, and the superficial and deep veins, which are beneficial to the establishment of the collateral circulation.

The veins with special structures include the **sinus of dura mater** (硬脑膜窦) and the **diploic vein** (板障静脉). The sinus of dura mater is located in the brain, which does not have the smooth muscle and valves. The diploic vein is located in the diploe, whose wall is thin and has no venous valves.

4.1   Pulmonary Veins

There are two pulmonary veins on each side, and they are called the **left superior pulmonary vein** (左上肺静脉), the **left inferior pulmonary vein** (左下肺静脉), the **right superior pulmonary vein** (右上肺静脉), and the **right inferior pulmonary vein** (右下肺静脉). The pulmonary veins arise from the hilum of the lungs, and enter the posterior part of the left atrium of the heart. The pulmonary veins carry the oxygenated blood from the lungs back to the left atrium. The left superior pulmonary vein and the left inferior pulmonary vein collect the blood from the upper and lower lobes of the left lung, respectively. The right superior pulmonary vein collects the blood from the upper and the middle lobes of the right lung; and the right inferior pulmonary vein collects the blood from the lower lobe of the right lung.

4.2   Systemic Veins

The systemic veins include the superior vena cava system, the inferior vena cava system, and the veins of the heart. Among the tributaries of inferior vena cava, the veins that collect the blood from unpaired organs (excluding the liver) are called the hepatic portal venous system.

4.2.1 Superior Vena Cava System

The **superior vena cava** (上腔静脉) and its tributaries collect the venous blood from the head, neck, upper limbs, and the chest (in addition to the heart and the lungs).

4.2.1.1   Veins of the head and neck

The superficial veins include the **facial vein** (面静脉), the **retromandibular vein** (下颌后静脉), the **anterior jugular vein** (颈前静脉), and the **external jugular vein** (颈外静脉). The deep veins include the **internal jugular vein** (颈内静脉), the **subclavian vein** (锁骨下静脉), and so on (Fig. 4-1).

1) Facial vein: The location of the facial vein is superficial. It arises from the angular vein, and descends behind the facial artery. It crosses the surface of the internal and external carotid arteries below the mandibular angle, and then enters the internal jugular vein near the greater horn of the hyoid bone. The facial vein communicates with the cavernous sinus through

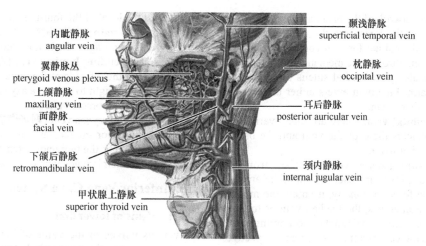

内眦静脉
angular vein

翼静脉丛
pterygoid venous plexus

上颌静脉
maxillary vein

面静脉
facial vein

下颌后静脉
retromandibular vein

甲状腺上静脉
superior thyroid vein

颞浅静脉
superficial temporal vein

枕静脉
occipital vein

耳后静脉
posterior auricular vein

颈内静脉
internal jugular vein

Figure 4-1 Veins of the head and neck.

the superior and the inferior ophthalmic veins. In another way, the facial vein communicates with the pterygoid plexus through the deep facial vein, and then communicates with the cavernous sinus.

2) Retromandibular vein: It is formed by the superficial temporal vein and the maxillary vein in the parotid gland. The maxillary vein arises from the pterygoid venous plexus located between the medial and lateral pterygoid muscles. At the lower end of the parotid gland, the retromandibular vein divides into the anterior and posterior branches. The anterior branch enters the facial vein, while the posterior branch anastomoses with the posterior auricular vein and the occipital vein to form the external jugular vein.

3) External jugular vein: It is formed by the posterior branch of the retromandibular vein, the posterior auricular vein, and the occipital vein at the place of the mandibular angle. It descends along the surface of the sternocleidomastoid muscle, piercing the deep fascia and entering either the subclavian vein or the venous angle.

4) Anterior jugular vein: The two anterior jugular veins descend on the two lateral sides of the median line of the neck, and finally enter the end of the external jugular veins or the subclavian veins. Above the manubrium sterni, the left and right anterior jugular veins anastomose with each other to form the jugular venous arch.

5) Internal jugular vein: It arises from the sigmoid sinus at the jugular foramen of the skull. In the carotid sheath, the internal jugular vein descends alongside the lateral side of the internal carotid artery and the common carotid artery, and then anastomoses with the subclavian vein to form the brachiocephalic vein behind the sternoclavicular joint.

6) Subclavian vein: It is the continuation of the axillary vein at the lateral border of the first rib, which runs under and forward of the axillary artery. Finally, it anastomoses with the internal jugular vein to form

the brachiocephalic vein behind the sternoclavicular joint, and the junction part is called thevenous angle.

4.2.1.2 Veins of upper limb

The superficial veins of the upper limb include the **cephalic vein** (头静脉), the **basilic vein** (贵要静脉), the **median cubital vein** (肘正中静脉), and the **median antebrachial vein** (前臂正中静脉) (Fig. 4-2).

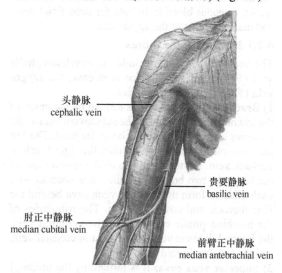

头静脉
cephalic vein

贵要静脉
basilic vein

肘正中静脉
median cubital vein

前臂正中静脉
median antebrachial vein

Figure 4-2 Superficial veins of the upper limb.

1) Cephalic vein: It originates from the radial side of the dorsal venous network of the hand. The cephalic vein ascends along the radial side of the forearm, the upper part of the forearm, the anterior surface of the elbow, and the lateral sulcus of the biceps branchii; it then reaches the subclavian fossa through the groove between the deltoid and the pectoralis major muscles. Finally, the cephalic vein enters either the axillary vein or the subclavian vein. It communicates with the basilic vein through the median cubital vein at the cubital fossa.

2) Basilic vein: It begins from the ulnar side of the

dorsal venous network of the hand, and ascends along the ulnar side of the forearm to the anterior aspect of the elbow. In the cubital fossa, it communicates with the cephalic vein through the median cubital vein, and then ascends along the medial sulcus to the middle level of the arm. Finally, it enters either the brachial vein or the axillary vein.

3) Median cubital vein: There are many variations; it usually connects the cephalic vein and the basilic vein in the cubital fossa.

4) Median antebrachial vein: It arises from the palmar venous plexus and ascends along the anterior surface of the forearm. Finally, it enters the median cubital vein. Sometimes, the median vein of forearm can be divided into two branches to communicate with the cephalic vein and the basilic vein, respectively. Therefore, under this situation, there is no median cubital vein.

The deep veins of the upper limb usually accompany their corresponding arteries. They have the same name and same course. However, there are usually two deep veins, such as the **brachial veins** (肱静脉). The two brachial veins to form the **axillary vein** (腋静脉) at the lower margin of the teres major muscle, and the axillary vein becomes the subclavian vein at the outer edge of the first rib. The axillary vein collects the venous blood from both the superficial veins and the deep veins of the upper limb.

4.2.1.3 Veins of the thorax

The veins of the thorax include the **brachiocephalic vein** (头臂静脉), the superior vena cava, the **azygos vein** (奇静脉) and its tributaries.

1) Brachiocephalic vein: It is formed by the union of the internal jugular vein and the subclavian vein at the posterior aspect of the sternoclavicular joint. The left brachiocephalic vein is longer than the right brachiocephalic vein. On the right side of the median line of the body, the two brachiocephalic veins connect with each other to form the superior vena cava behind the first thoracic and costal junction. The tributaries of the brachiocephalic vein include the vertebral vein, the internal thoracic vein, the highest intercostal vein, and the inferior thyroid vein.

2) Superior vena cava: It is formed by the union of the left and right brachiocephalic veins. The superior vena cava descends along the right side of the ascending aorta; it passes through the fibrous pericardium at the posterior aspect of the right second sternocostal joint, and finally enters the right atrium at the lower border of the third sternocostal joint. Before it passes through the fibrous pericardium, the azygos vein enters the superior vena cava.

3) Azygos vein: At the place of the right crural diaphragm, the azygos vein arises from the **right ascending lumbar vein** (右腰升静脉). It ascends along the posterior surface of the esophagus and the right side of the thoracic aorta, and then enters the superior vena cava at the level of the fourth thoracic vertebra.

4) Hemiazygos vein (半奇静脉)**:** At the place of the left crural diaphragm, the hemiazygos vein arises from the **left ascending lumbar vein** (左腰升静脉). It ascends along the left side of the thoracic vertebrae, and then turns the right to enter the azygos vein at the level of the eighth thoracic vertebra.

5) Accessory hemiazygos vein (副半奇静脉)**:** It arises from the posterior intercostal veins and descends along the left side of the thoracic vertebrae. Finally, it enters either the hemiazygos vein or the azygos vein.

4.2.2 Inferior Vena Cava System

4.2.2.1 Veins of lower limb

The venous valves in the veins of lower limb are more than that of the upper limb, and the traffic branches between the superficial veins and deep veins are also rich. The superficial veins and deep veins of the lower limb include the small saphenous vein, the great saphenous vein, the anterior and posterior tibial veins, the popliteal vein, and the femoral vein.

1) Small saphenous vein (小隐静脉)**:** It begins from the dorsal venous arch of the foot at the lateral margin of foot. The small saphenous vein ascends along the posterior surface of the leg, passing through the posterior aspect of the lateral ankle, and then runs between the two heads of the gastrocnemius. Finally, it enters the popliteal vein.

2) Great saphenous vein (大隐静脉)**:** It is the longest vein in the human body, which arises from the dorsal venous arch of the foot at the medial margin of foot. After crossing the anterior aspect of the medial ankle, the great saphenous vein ascends along the medial side of the leg, the posterior surface of the knee, and the medial side of the thigh to the saphenous hiatus. Finally, it enters the femoral vein. Before the great saphenous vein enters the femoral vein, it accepts the **superficial epigastric vein** (腹壁浅动脉), the **superficial iliac circumflex vein** (旋髂浅静脉), the **external pudendal vein** (阴部外静脉), the **superficial medial femoral vein** (股内侧浅静脉), and the **superficial lateral femoral vein** (股外侧浅静脉) (Fig. 4-3).

The deep veins of the foot and leg accompany their corresponding arteries, which have the same names and the same courses. The **popliteal vein** (腘静脉) is formed by the **anterior and posterior tibial veins** (胫前、后静脉), and the **femoral vein** (股静脉) is the direct continuation of the popliteal vein. The femoral vein accompanying the femoral artery becomes the external iliac vein after it passes through the inguinal ligament.

4.2.2.2 Veins of the abdominal and pelvic region

The veins of the abdominal and pelvic region include the external iliac vein, the internal iliac vein, the inferior vena cava, and the hepatic portal vein and its

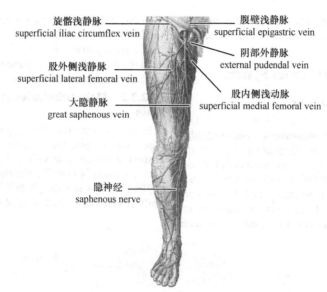

旋髂浅静脉
superficial iliac circumflex vein

股外侧浅静脉
superficial lateral femoral vein

大隐静脉
great saphenous vein

隐神经
saphenous nerve

腹壁浅静脉
superficial epigastric vein

阴部外静脉
external pudendal vein

股内侧浅动脉
superficial medial femoral vein

Figure 4-3　The great saphenous vein.

tributaries.

1) External iliac vein (髂外静脉): It is the direct continuation of the femoral vein. The left external iliac vein ascends along the medial side of the left external iliac artery, while the right iliac vein ascends along the medial side of the right external iliac artery first, and then ascends along the posterior surface of the right external iliac artery. The two external iliac veins connect with each other to form the common iliac vein in front of the sacroiliac joint. The external iliac vein accepts the **inferior epigastric vein (腹壁下静脉)** and the **deep iliac circumflex vein (旋髂深静脉)**.

2) Internal iliac vein (髂内静脉): The two internal iliac veins ascend along the internal iliac artery, and then connect with the corresponding arteries to form the common iliac veins, respectively. The tributaries of the internal iliac vein accompany their corresponding arteries, and the veins form the rich venous plexus on the surface of the abdominal and pelvic organs. In male, there are the **vesical venous plexus (膀胱静脉丛)** and **rectal venous plexus (直肠静脉丛)**. In addition to these, there are also the **uterine venous plexus (子宫静脉脉丛)** and **vaginal venous plexus (阴道静脉丛)** in female.

3) Common iliac vein (髂总静脉): It is formed by the fusion of external and internal iliac veins. The two common iliac veins accompany the corresponding common iliac arteries and form the inferior vena cava at the right side of the fifth lumbar vertebra. The left common iliac vein is long and tilted; it ascends along the medial side of the left common iliac artery first, and then ascends along the posterior aspect of the right common iliac artery. The right common iliac vein is short and vertical; it ascends along the posterior aspect of the right common iliac artery, and then ascends along the lateral side of the right common

iliac artery. The two common iliac veins accept the **iliolumbar veins (髂腰静脉)** and the **lateral sacral veins (骶外侧静脉)**, and the left common iliac vein also accepts the **median sacral vein (骶正中静脉)**.

4) Inferior vena cava (下腔静脉): It ascends along the right side of the abdominal aorta, passes through the sulcus of vena cava and enters the thoracic cavity through the vena cava foramen, and then enters the right atrium through the fibrous pericardium. The tributaries of the inferior vena cava include the parietal tributaries and the visceral tributaries, and most of them accompany the corresponding arteries.

The parietal tributaries include a pair of **inferior phrenic veins (膈下静脉)** and 4 pairs of **lumbar veins (腰静脉)**. The vertical tributaries between the lumbar veins form the ascending lumbar vein, and the left and right ascending lumbar veins form the hemiazygos vein and azygos vein, respectively.

The visceral tributaries include the **testicular vein (睾丸静脉)** or the **ovarian vein (卵巢静脉)**, the **renal vein (肾静脉)**, the **suprarenal vein (肾上腺静脉)** and the **hepatic vein (肝静脉)**.

The testicular vein arises from the pampiniform plexus, which is formed by the anastomosis of the small veins of the testis and epididymis. The ovarian vein arises from the ovarian venous plexus, which ascends in the suspensory ligament of the ovary.

The veins of the kidney connect with each other to form a single trunk at the place of the renal hilum. The renal vein runs in front of the renal artery and finally enters the inferior vena cava. The left renal vein is longer than the right renal vein, which crosses the anterior surface of the abdominal aorta. The left renal vein accepts the left testicular vein and left suprarenal vein.

The left suprarenal vein enters the left renal vein, and the right suprarenal vein enters the inferior vena cava.

The left, middle, and right hepatic veins enter the inferior vena cava at the place of the sulcus of vena cava.

4.2.3　Hepatic Portal Venous System

4.2.3.1　Hepatic portal vein

The **hepatic portal vein** (肝门静脉) (Fig. 4-4) is formed by the **superior mesenteric vein** (肠系膜上静脉) and the **splenic vein** (脾静脉) at the posterior aspect of the neck of the pancreas. It ascends between the neck of the pancreas and the inferior vena cava to enter the hepatoduodenal ligament, and then ascends along the posterior aspect of the proper hepatic artery and common bile duct to reach the porta of the liver.

Finally, it divides into two tributaries to enter the left and right lobes of the liver, respectively. The blood of the hepatic portal vein flows into the hepatic sinusoid, and the blood from the hepatic sinusoid flows into the inferior vena cava through the hepatic veins.

4.2.3.2　Main tributaries of the hepatic portal vein

The main tributaries of the hepatic portal vein include the splenic vein, the superior mesenteric vein, the **inferior mesenteric vein** (肠系膜下静脉), the **left gastric vein** (胃左静脉), the **right gastric vein** (胃右静脉), the **cystic vein** (胆囊静脉), and the **paraumbilical vein** (附脐静脉) (Fig. 4-4).

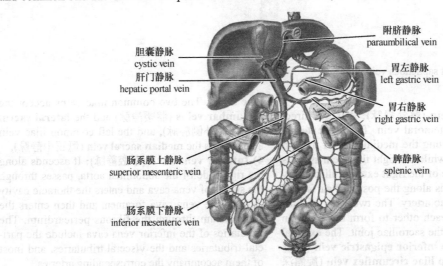

Figure 4-4　Main tributaries of the hepatic portal vein.

The splenic vein arises from the porta of the spleen, which connects with the superior mesenteric vein to form the hepatic portal vein. The inferior mesenteric vein enters the splenic vein or superior mesenteric vein. The left gastric vein anastomoses with the tributaries of the azygos vein and hemiazygos vein. The right gastric vein accepts the **prepyloric vein** (幽门前静脉). The cystic vein enters the trunk or the right branch of the hepatic portal vein. The paraumbilical vein arises from the periumbilical venous rete, which can be divided into two tributaries to enter the hepatic portal vein.

4.2.3.3　Anastomoses between the hepatic portal venous system and the vena caval system

1) Esophageal venous plexus (食管静脉丛): The left gastric vein of the hepatic portal venous system communicates with the azygos vein and hemiazygos vein of the superior vena cava system through the esophageal venous plexus.

2) Rectal venous plexus (直肠静脉丛): The superior rectal vein of the hepatic portal venous system communicates with the inferior rectal vein and the anal vein of the inferior vena cava system through the rectal venous plexus.

3) Periumbilical venous rete (脐周静脉网): The paraumbilical vein of the hepatic portal venous system communicates with the thoraco-epigastric vein and the superior epigastric vein of the superior vena cava system through the periumbilical venous rete. The paraumbilical vein of the hepatic portal venous system communicates with the superficial epigastric vein and inferior epigastric vein of the inferior vena cava system through the periumbilical venous rete.

4) Internal and external vertebral venous plexus (椎内、外静脉丛): The small veins of the hepatic portal venous system communicate with the posterior intercostal veins and lumbar veins of the superior and inferior vena cava sytems through the internal and external vertebral venous plexus.

Summary

静脉是运送血液回心的血管，起于毛细血管，止于心房。数量比动脉多，具有静脉瓣，以保证血液向心流动和防止血液逆流。

肺静脉是从肺输送含氧量较高的动脉血注入左心房，每侧两条，分别为左上、左下肺静脉和右上、右下肺静脉。

体循环静脉分为浅静脉和深静脉，包括上腔静脉系、下腔静脉系和心静脉系，其上腔静脉系由上腔静脉及其属支组成，收集头颈部、上肢和胸部（心、肺除外）等上半身的静脉血。下腔静脉系由下腔静脉及其属支组成收集下半身的静脉血，其中由肝门静脉及其属支组成，收集腹盆部消化道、脾、胰和胆囊的静脉血，起始端和末端分别与毛细血管相连，无瓣膜。

在静脉知识的学习中，由于深静脉多与同名动脉伴行，故只要良好的掌握了动脉的知识，就会对人体全身的深静脉具有基础性的掌握。因此，静脉中的浅静脉是学生学习的重点。

Jin Haifeng, Wang Lulu (金海峰，王璐璐)

Part II Cardiovascular Histology

Chapter 5 The Histological Structure of Circulatory System

The circulatory system comprises two systems: the blood and lymphatic vascular systems. The blood vascular system is composed of the heart, arteries, veins and capillaries. The heart can pump the blood and make the blood flow in blood vessels. The arteries are a series of efferent vessels that become smaller as they branch, and the function of the arteries is to carry the blood which is full of nutrients and oxygen to the tissues. The capillaries are the smallest blood vessels. The capillaries anastomose profusely and constitute a complex network. The interchange between blood and tissues takes place through the walls of the capillaries. The capillaries converge to the veins. The veins become larger when they approach the heart, toward which they convey the blood to be pumped again.

The lymphatic vascular system begins in the lymphatic capillaries. The lymphatic capillaries are closed-ended tubules and the tubules can anastomose to form vessels of steadily increasing size; these vessels mingle in the blood vascular system emptying into the large veins near the heart. One of the functions of the lymphatic system is to absorb the fluid from the tissue spaces to the blood. The internal surface of all sections of the blood and lymphatic systems is covered by a single layer of a squamous epithelium, called **endothelium** (内皮).

5.1 Capillaries

The number of the capillary network depends on the metabolic activity of the tissues. Tissues with high metabolic rates have an abundant capillary network, such as the kidney, liver, and cardiac and skeletal muscle. On the contrary, in the tissues with low metabolic rates, such as **smooth muscle** (平滑肌) and **dense connective tissue** (致密结缔组织), there are very few capillaries.

5.1.1 General Structure

Capillaries have structural variations to allow exchange of different materials between blood and surrounding tissues. Capillaries are composed of a single layer of endothelial cells. The average diameter of capillaries is 7–9μm and the longest capillary is about 50μm. The total length of capillaries in the human body is estimated to be 96,000km (60,000miles). In the cross-section, the walls of capillaries consist of portions of 1–3 cells (Fig. 5-1). The external surfaces of these cells usually attach on a **basal lamina** (基

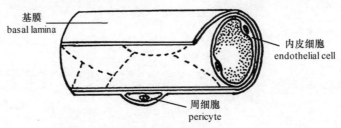

基膜
basal lamina

内皮细胞
endothelial cell

周细胞
pericyte

Figure 5-1 The structure of a capillary with fenestrae in its wall.

板) which is produced by the endothelial cells. There are **pericytes** (周细胞) between the basal lamina and the endothelial cells. The function of pericytes is not known now.

Observing from the surface, endothelial cells are usual polygonal and elongated in the direction of blood flow. The nuclei of the cells bulge into the capillary lumen. In its **cytoplasm** (细胞质), there are a few organelles, including a small **Golgi complex** (高尔基复合体), free **ribosomes** (核糖体), **mitochondria** (线粒体) and a few cisternae of **rough endoplasmic reticulum** (粗面内质网) (Fig. 5-2). Between most endothelial cells, junctions of the **zonula occludens** (闭锁小带) type are present and are import-

ant for physiology.

Surrounding the endothelial cells, there are mesenchymal origin cells at various locations along the capillaries and the postcapillary venules. These cells are called pericytes, and have long cytoplasmic processes.

They are between their own basal lamina and the endothelial cells. **Myosin** (肌球蛋白), **actin** (肌动蛋白) and **tropomyosin** (原肌球蛋白) are present in pericytes, which strongly suggest that these cells also have a contractile function. After tissue injurieed, the pericytes may participate in the repair process by proliferating and differentiating to form new blood vessels and connective tissue cells.

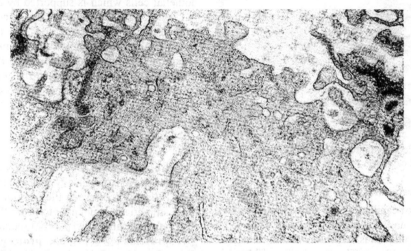

Figure 5-2　Electron micrograph of a section of a continuous capillary.

5.1.2　Classification

Blood capillaries can be grouped into 3 types, depending on the continuity of both the basal lamina and the endothelial sheet.

5.1.2.1　Continuous Capillary

The character of **continuous capillary** (连续毛细血管) (Fig. 5-3) is that its wall is absent of fenestrae. This type of capillary is found in all kinds of connective tissue, muscle tissue, nervous tissue and exocrine glands. Except for the nervous system, on both surfaces of the endothelial cells numerous **pinocytotic vesicles** (吞饮小泡) can be observed. Pinocytotic vesicles are also present as isolated vesicles in the cytoplasm of these cells and are responsible for the transport of **macromolecules** (大分子物质) directly across the endothelial cytoplasm.

5.1.2.2　Fenestrated Capillary

The **fenestrated capillaries** (有孔毛细血管) are characterized by the presence of large fenestrae in the walls of endothelial cells. Some of the fenestrae are obliterated by a diaphragm that does not have the trilaminar structure of a unit membrane. So it is thinner

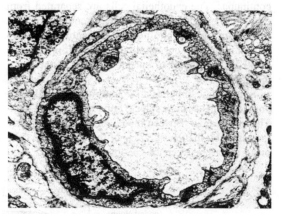

Figure 5-3　Electron micrograph of a transverse section of a continuous capillary.

than a cell membrane (Fig. 5-1, Fig. 5-4). The basal lamina of the fenestrated capillaries is continuous. Fenestrated capillaries are found in tissues of the kidney, intestine and endocrine glands. In these organs, interchange of substances between the tissues and the blood is very fast, macromolecules can cross the endothelial cells through the fenestrae and then cross the basal lamina into the tissue spaces. There is a special kind of fenestrated capillary. It is characteristic of the renal glomerulus. These fenestrae of the capillaries are devoid of diaphragm. In this type of capillary, the blood is separated from the tissues only by a continuous and very thick basal lamina that surrounds the fenestrae.

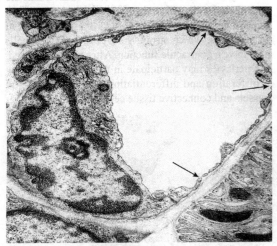

Figure 5-4 Electron micrograph of a transverse section of a fenestrated capillary.

5.1.2.3 Sinusoidal Capillary

The last type of capillary is the **sinusoidal capillary** (血窦), which has the following characteristics: The path of the capillaries is serpentine and the diameter gets larger (30–40μm). The circulation of blood is slower in these capillaries. The basal lamina is discontinuous. The endothelial cells are separated from each other by wide spaces and are discontinuous. The cytoplasm of the endothelial cells shows multiple fenestrations without diaphragms. Macrophages are located either among or outside the cells of the endothelium.

Sinusoidal capillaries are found mainly in hematopoietic organs such as spleen, bone marrow and liver. The interchange between blood and tissues is greatly facilitated by the fenestrations of the endothelial cells or the spaces between the endothelial cells.

5.2 Structural Features of Blood Vessels

All blood vessels above a certain diameter have a lot of structural features in common and present a general plan of construction. However, the same type of vessels can show obvious structural variations. On the other hand, the difference between diverse types is often not clear-cut because the transition from one vessel type to another is gradual.

5.2.1 Tunica Intima

The **tunica intima** (内膜) displays one layer of endothelial cells which is supported by a subendothelial layer of loose connective tissue containing few smooth muscle cells. In arteries, the outer layer of the intima is the internal elastic membrane, which separates the intima from the media. There are gaps (fenestrae) made of elastin in the internal elastic membrane, allowing the material to diffuse to the cells deep into the wall of the blood vessel. (Fig. 5-6, Fig. 5-10).

5.2.2 Tunica Media

The **tunica media** (中膜) is mainly composed of concentric layers of helically arranged smooth muscle cells (Fig. 5-6). Between the smooth muscle cells, there are variable amounts of **elastic fibers** (弹性纤维), **reticular fibers** (网状纤维) (collagen type Ⅲ), **glycoproteins** (糖蛋白), and **proteoglycans** (蛋白多糖). Smooth muscle cells are the cellular source of this extracellular matrix. In some arteries, there is a thinner external elastic membrane, which separates the tunica media from the adventitia.

5.2.3 Adventitia

The **adventitia** (外膜) consists principally of elastic and type Ⅰ collagen fibers (Fig. 5-5, Fig. 5-6). When the vessel goes through the organ, the adventitial layer gradually becomes continuous with the surrounding connective tissue.

In the adventitia and the outer part of the media of

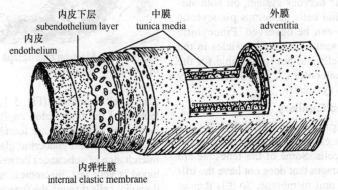

内皮下层
subendothelium layer

中膜
tunica media

外膜
adventitia

内皮
endothelium

内弹性膜
internal elastic membrane

Figure 5-5 A medium-sized muscular artery.

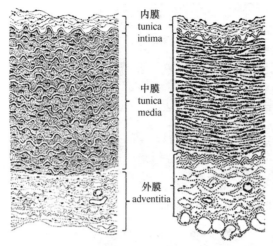

内膜
tunica
intima

中膜
tunica
media

外膜
adventitia

Figure 5-6 Diagrams of an elastic artery (left) and a muscular artery (right).

the large vessels, **vasa vasorum** (营养血管) ("vessels of the vessel"), which are arterioles, capillaries and venules, is usually present. The vasa vasorum nourishes the adventitia and the media, since the layers are too thick in larger vessels and hardly get nutrients solely by diffusion from the blood in the lumen. Vasa vasorum is more often present in veins than in ar-

teries (Fig. 5-6, Fig. 5-11). In intermediate and large arteries, there is no vasa vasorum in the intima and the most internal region of the media. These layers receive oxygen and nutrients by diffusion from the blood that circulates into the lumen of the vessel.

5.3 Arteries

The arterial blood vessels are classified into arteries of medium diameter (muscular arteries) and larger (elastic) arteries according to their diameter.

5.3.1 Arterioles

The diameter of **arterioles** (微动脉) is generally less than 0.5mm, and lumen is relatively narrow (Fig. 5-7, Fig. 5-13). The subendothelial layer is very thin. There is no internal elastic membrane in the very small arterioles, and the media is generally composed of one or two circularly arranged layers of smooth muscle cells; it shows no external elastic membrane (Fig. 5-7, Fig. 5-13). Above the arterioles are small arteries. The tunica media of small arteries is more developed, and the lumen is larger than those of the arterioles (Fig. 5-8, Fig. 5-9, Fig. 5-10). The tunica adventitia is very thin in both arterioles and small arteries.

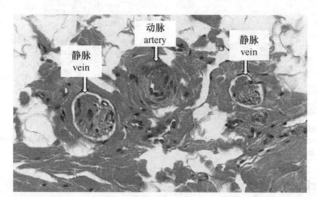

Figure 5-7 Cross section through an arteriole and its accompanying venule from the myometrium of mouse uterus.

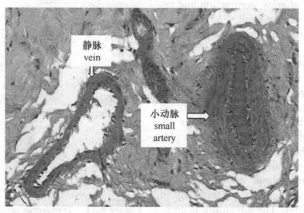

Figure 5-8 Cross section through a small artery and its accompanying muscular vein.

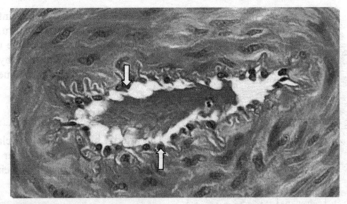

Figure 5-9   A small artery. The endothelial layer covering the lumen of the vessel.

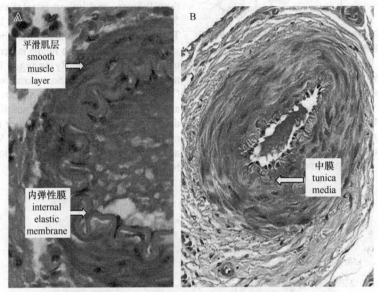

平滑肌层
smooth
muscle
layer

内弹性膜
internal
elastic
membrane

中膜
tunica
media

Figure 5-10   Cross sections of small arteries.
A: The elastic lamina is not stained and is seen as a pallid lamina of scalloped appearance just below the endothelium (arrowhead). B: A small artery with a distinctly stained internal elastic membrane.

5.3.2 Medium Arteries

Medium arteries (中动脉) are also named muscular arteries. In the muscular arteries, contraction and relaxation of the smooth muscle cells in the tunica media can control the affluence of blood flowing to the organ. The intima has a subendothelial layer that is thicker than that of the arterioles (Fig. 5-5, Fig. 5-11). The **internal elastic membrane** (内弹性膜), which is the most external component of the intima, is obvious (Fig. 5-11), and the tunica media may contain up to 40 layers of smooth muscle cells. These cells are mixed with various numbers of elastic lamellae (depending on the size of the vessel) as well as proteoglycans and reticular fibers, all made by the smooth muscle fibers. The external elastic membrane is the last component of the media, and is present only in the larger muscular arteries. The adventitia is composed of connective tissue. Vasa vasorum, nerves, and

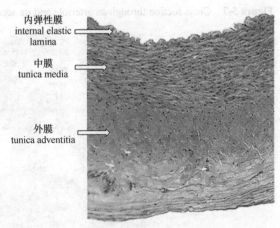

内弹性膜
internal elastic
lamina

中膜
tunica media

外膜
tunica adventitia

Figure 5-11   Transverse section showing part of a muscular (medium caliber) artery.

lymphatic capillaries are also found in the adventitia, and these structures may penetrate to the outer part of the media.

5.3.3 Large Arteries

Large arteries (大动脉) are also named elastic arteries. The blood flows stably in large arteries. The elastic arteries include the aorta and its large branches. They have a yellowish color from the accumulation of elastin in the media (Fig. 5-6, Fig. 5-12). The intima is thicker than the corresponding layer of a muscular artery. The internal elastic membrane is present, but is not easily discerned, since it is similar to the elastic membranes in the next layer. The media is composed of elastic fibers and a series of concentrically perforated, arranged elastic membranes whose number increases with age (there are 40 in the newborn, 70 in the adult). Between the elastic membranes, there are smooth muscle cells, proteoglycans, glycoproteins and reticular fibers. The adventitia is relatively underdeveloped.

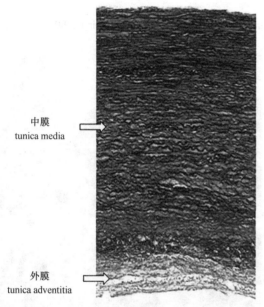

中膜
tunica media

外膜
tunica adventitia

Figure 5-12 Transverse section showing part of a large elastic artery with a well developed tunica media containing several elastic laminas.

The several elastic membranes have the function of making the blood outflow more uniform. When the ventricle contracts, the elastic membranes of large arteries are stretched and reduce changes of pressure. During ventricular relaxation, ventricular pressure drops to a low level. But the elastic rebound of large arteries helps maintain arterial pressure. As a result, blood velocity and arterial pressure become less variable as the distance from the heart increases.

5.4 Veins

5.4.1 Venules and Postcapillary Venules

The diameter of **venules** (微静脉) is 0.2 to 1mm. Their tunica intima is composed of endothelium and a very thin subendothelial layer. In small venules, the media may contain only contractile pericytes. These vessels are called **postcapillary venules** (毛细血管后微静脉). Their luminal diameter is more than 50μm. However, most venules are muscular, with at least a few smooth muscle cells in their walls (Fig. 5-7, Fig. 5-16). Postcapillary venules have several features in common with capillaries, e.g., participation in the exchange of cells and molecules between blood and tissues and inflammatory processes. Junctions between endothelial cells of venules are the loosest. At these locations, during the inflammatory response, fluid can escape from the circulatory system and lead to edema. Venules may also affect blood flow in the arterioles by producing and secreting diffusible vasoactive substances.

5.4.2 Medium-sized Veins

The diameters of majority **medium-sized or small veins** (中静脉或小静脉) are 1 to 9mm (Fig. 5-8, Fig. 5-13). The intima usually has a thin subendothelial layer, but sometimes it may be absent. The media is composed of small bundles of smooth muscle cells intermixed with reticular fibers and a delicate network of elastic fibers. The collagenous adventitial layer is well developed.

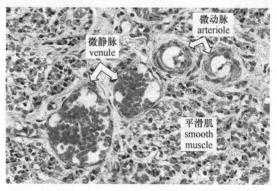

微动脉
arteriole

微静脉
venule

平滑肌
smooth
muscle

Figure 5-13 Cross section of 2 venules and 2 small arterioles.

5.4.3 Large Veins

The **large veins** (大静脉) are the major venous trunks which are close to the heart. Tunica intima of large veins is well-developed, but the media is much thinner, with abundant connective tissue and few layers of smooth muscle cells. The adventitial layer is the best-developed and thickest layer in veins; it often contains longitudinal bundles of smooth muscle (Fig.

5-14). These veins, especially the largest ones, have **valves** (瓣膜) in their interior (Fig. 5-15). The valves consist of 2 semilunar folds of the tunica intima which project into the lumen. They are composed of connective tissue which are rich in elastic fibers and are lined on both sides by endothelium. The valves, which are particularly numerous in veins of the limbs, direct the venous blood toward the heart. The propulsive force of the heart is reinforced by contraction of skeletal muscles that surround these veins.

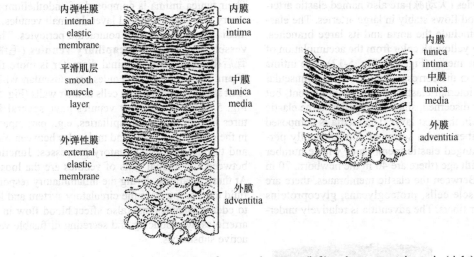

Figure 5-14　Diagram comparing the structure of a muscular artery (left) and accompanying vein (right).

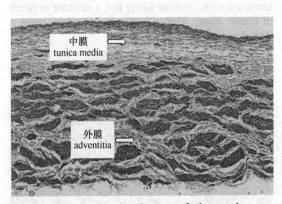

Figure 5-15　Section showing part of a large vein.

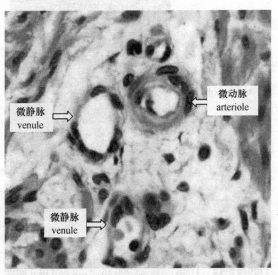

Figure 5-16　Small blood vessels from the microvasculature.

5.5　Heart

5.5.1　Wall of Heart

The heart is a muscular organ that contracts rhythmically, pumping the blood through the circulatory system. It also produces a hormone called atrial natriuretic factor. Its walls consist of 3 layers: **endocardium** (心内膜), **myocardium** (心肌膜), **epicardium** (心外膜). The fibrous central region of the heart, called the fibrous skeleton, serves as the base of the valves and the site of origin and insertion of the cardiac muscle cells.

The endocardium is homologous with the intima of blood vessels. It is composed of a single layer of squamous endothelial cells and a thin **subendothelial layer** (内皮下层) of loose connective tissue that contains some smooth muscle cells, collagen and elastic fibers. A layer of connective tissue, which is often called the **subendocardial layer** (心内膜下层), connects the myocardium to the subendothelial layer. The subendocardial layer contains veins, nerves and branches of the impulse-conducting system of the heart which are called Purkinje fibers.

The myocardium is the thickest layer of the heart. It consists of cardiac muscle cells arranging in layers that surround the heart chambers in a complex spiral. A large number of these layers insert themselves into the fibrous **cardiac skeleton** (心骨骼). The arrangement of these muscle cells is extremely varied, so that cells are seen to be oriented in many directions in histological sections of a small area. The heart is covered externally by simple squamous epithelium which is called **mesothelium** (间皮) supported by a thin layer of connective tissue that constitutes the epicardium. The layer of loose connective tissue contains nerves, **nerve ganglia** (神经节), and veins. The **adipose tissue** (脂肪组织) that generally surrounds the heart accumulates in this layer. The epicardium corresponds to the visceral layer of the pericardium, the serous membrane in which the heart lies. There is a small amount of fluid between the visceral layer and the parietal layer that facilitates the heart's movements.

The cardiac skeleton consists of dense connective tissue. Its principal components are the trigonal fibrosa, the annuli fibrosa, and the septum membranaceum. These structures are composed of dense connective tissue, with thick collagen fibers oriented in various directions. Certain regions contain nodules of fibrous cartilage.

The **cardiac valves** (心瓣膜) are composed of a central core of dense fibrous connective tissue (containing both elastic and collagen fibers), lined on both sides by endothelial layers. The bases of the valves are attached to the annuli fibrosa of the fibrous skeleton.

5.5.2 Conducting System of the Heart

The heart has a specialized system to form a rhythmic stimulus which is spread to the entire myocardium. This system (Fig. 5-17, Fig. 5-18) which is called the conducting system of the heart, consists of 2 nodes located in the atrium, the atrioventricular node and sinoatrial node, and by the atrioventricular bundle. The atrioventricular bundle originates from the node of the same name and branches to both ventricles. The cells of the impulse-conducting system are function-

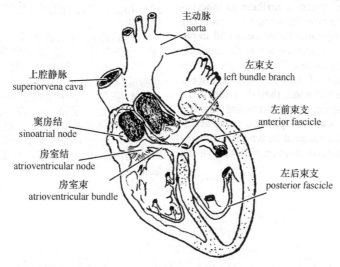

Figure 5-17   Diagram of the heart, showing the impulse-generating and-conducting system.

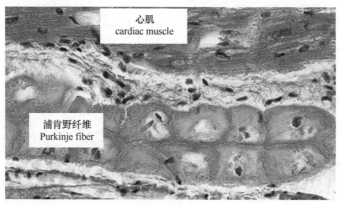

Figure 5-18   Purkinje cells of the impulse-conducting system.

ally integrated by gap junctions. The sinoatrial node consists of a large number of modified cardiac muscle cells that are fusiform, have fewer myofibrils, and are smaller than atrial muscle cells. The cells of the atrioventricular node are similar to those of the sinoatrial node, but their cytoplasmic projections branch in different directions, forming a network.

The atrioventricular bundle is formed by cells similar to those of the atrioventricular node. Distally, however, these cells become larger than ordinary cardiac muscle cells and have a distinctive appearance. These cells which are called Purkinje fibers have one or two central nuclei, and their cytoplasm is rich in glycogen and mitochondria. The myofibrils are sparse and only found in the periphery of the cytoplasm (Fig. 5-18). After traveling through the subendocardial layer, they penetrate the ventricles and sinuses become endocardium. This arrangement is very important for the stimulus getting into the innermost layers of the ventricular musculature.

5.5.3　Innervation

Both the sympathetic and parasympathetic divisions of nervous autonomic system contribute to innervation of the heart and form widespread plexuses at the base of the heart. Ganglionic nerve cells and nerve fibers are present in the regions close to the sinoatrial and atrioventricular nodes. Though these nerves do not affect formation of the heartbeat, a process attributed to the sinoatrial node, they do affect heart rhythm, such as during emotional stress and physical exercise. Stimulation of the sympathetic nerve accelerates the rhythm of the pacemaker, whereas stimulation of the parasympathetic division slows down the heartbeat.

Between the muscular fibers of the myocardium, there are a lot of afferent free nerve endings which are related to sensibility and pain. Partial obstruction of the coronary arteries reduces the supply of oxygen to the myocardium and causes pain. The same sensorial enervation happens on a heart attack, which is very painful because many muscular fibers die from the low levels of oxygen.

Summary

心血管系统除毛细血管外都存在着共同的结构。血管壁可分三层：内膜、中膜和外膜。心脏壁的三层称为心内膜、心肌膜和心外膜。

毛细血管的结构最简单，仅由一层内皮细胞、基膜和周细胞组成，周细胞的胞质突起较长，部分围绕着内皮细胞。毛细血管可分为连续毛细血管、有孔毛细血管和血窦三种。

动脉可按其大小分为四种：大动脉、中动脉、小动脉和微动脉。由于动脉的大小和相应结构的变化通常是渐进的，因此在不同的动脉之间存在着明确的界限。大动脉属于弹性动脉。人体内大部分命名的动脉属于中动脉，其中膜有10~40层密集排列的平滑肌细胞，因此被称为肌性动脉。

与其相应的动脉相比，静脉管腔大，管壁薄。由于静脉内、外弹力膜常缺失；外膜是静脉最厚的一层，许多静脉，尤其是四肢静脉，都设有静脉瓣，防止血液回流。

心脏是一个中空的肌性器官。心内膜分为内皮、内皮下层和心内膜下层。心内膜下层可见心脏传导系统的分支。心肌膜是心脏中最厚的一层，它有丰富的毛细血管供应。心肌细胞大致分为内纵行、中环行和外斜行三层。心外膜为浆膜。

Zhang Meng (张萌)

Part Ⅲ   Cardiovascular Physiology

Chapter 6   Overview of the Cardiovascular System

6.1 Cardiovascular System

The overall functional arrangement of the **cardiovascular system** (循环系统) is shown in Fig. 6-1. This figure shows the functional relationship of the heart and various organs rather than the anatomical relationship. The functional manifestations of the heart are mainly: the pumping function of the left ventricle and the right ventricle. Therefore, it is generally believed that the cardiovascular system includes the systemic circulation and the pulmonary circulation. Systemic circulation: arterial blood from the left ventricle→aorta→various organ arteries→capillary → various veins →superior vena cava/inferior vena cava→right atrium; pulmonary circulation: venous blood from the right ventricle→pulmonary trunk and its branches→alveolar capillary→pulmonary veins→left atrium. All blood flows through the pulmonary circulation and the systemic circulation is made up of many parallel connected vascular circulations. The vascular system of the systemic circulation and the pulmonary circulation is composed of the arteries, capillaries and veins which are connected in series, and the systemic circulation and the pulmonary circulation are also connected by the heart. Therefore, the left and right ventricles must be pumping out the same amount of blood every minute. The amount of blood pumped out of one ventricle per minute is called the **cardiac output** (CO, 心输出量). The normal value of cardiac output is 5–6L/min.

As indicated in Fig. 6-1, systemic organs are functionally parallel in the cardiovascular system. This parallel arrangement has two important implications. Firstly, nearly all of the systemic organs receive arterial blood, a highly oxygenated blood that has just passed through the pulmonary circulation. Secondly, the blood flow through any one of the systemic organs can be controlled independently. For example, during strenuous exercise, this cardiovascular reflex can occur: the blood flow to the muscle tissue increases, to the kidney decreases.

Because friction develops between the blood and the vascular walls and in the blood vessels, there's resistance to blood flow. Blood can overcome resistance of blood flow through the blood vessels in the organs simply because there is a pressure difference between the arteries and the veins. The main job of the heart pump is to keep the pressure in the arteries greater than the veins. Generally, the average pressure in systemic arteries is close to 100mmHg, and that of systemic veins is close to 0mmHg. Therefore, since the pressure differences between the arteries and the veins in all systemic organs are the same, cardiac output is distributed among the various systemic organs solely on the basis of their individual resistance to blood flow. Since blood flows along the path of least resistance, organs with relatively low resistance receive relatively high blood flow.

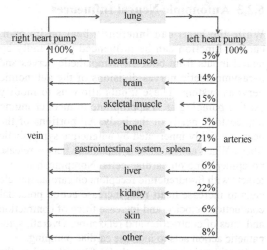

Figure 6-1 Percentage of cardiac output distributed in different organ systems in a quiet state.

6.2 Heart

The heart lies in the center of the pericardium. The pericardium is the conical fibrous serous capsule that encloses the heart and the roots of the great vessels. A small amount of fluid in the sac lubricates the surface of the heart and allows it to move freely during contraction and relaxation.

6.2.1 Pumping Action

Blood flow through all organs is passive and occurs only because the arterial pressure is kept higher than the venous pressure by the pumping action of the heart. The right heart pump provides the energy necessary to move blood through the pulmonary vessels, and the left heart pump provides the energy to move blood through the systemic organs.

The amount of blood from each ventricle pumped per minute (**CO**) depends on the volume of blood ejected per beat, the **stroke volume** (**SV**, 每搏输出量) and the number of heart beats per minute, **the heart rate** (**HR**, 心率) as follows:

$$CO = SV \times HR$$

It should be evident from this relationship that all influences on cardiac output must act by changing either the heart rate or the stroke volume.

Venous blood returns from the systemic organs to the right atrium via the superior and inferior vena cava. It passes through the tricuspid valve into the right ventricle and from there is pumped through the pulmonary valve into the pulmonary circulation via the pulmonary arteries. Oxygenated pulmonary venous blood flows in the pulmonary veins to the left atrium and passes through the mitral valve into the left ventricle. From there it is pumped through the aortic valve into the aorta to be distributed to the systemic organs.

Although the gross anatomy of the right heart pump is somewhat different from that of the left heart pump, the pumping principles are identical. The heart is divided into four chambers by the left atrioventricular valve and the right atrioventricular valve: left atrium, right atrium, left ventricle and right ventricle. The left ventricle and the aorta are separated by the aortic valve. The right ventricle and the pulmonary artery are separated by the pulmonary valve. Since both the atrioventricular and arterial valves are one-way open, these valves can only open when the pressure of the atrium is greater than the ventricles and the pressure of the ventricles is greater than the arteries, and the blood flows from the atrium to the ventricles and the arteries along the pressure gradient. Ventricular pumping occurs because the volume of the ventricle is periodically altered by the rhythm and synchronous contraction as well as the relaxation of ventricular muscle cells in the circumferential direction of the ventricle wall.

When the ventricular muscle cells are contracting, they generate a circumferential tension in the ventricular walls that causes the pressure within the chamber to increase. As soon as the ventricular pressure exceeds the pressure in the pulmonary artery (right pump) or the aorta (left pump), blood is forced out of the chamber through the outlet valve. This phase of the cardiac cycle during which the ventricular muscle cells are contracting is called the systole. Because the pressure is higher in the ventricle than in the atrium during systole, the inlet or atrioventricular valve is closed. When the ventricular muscle cells relax, the pressure in the ventricle falls below that in the atrium, the atrioventricular valve opens, and the ventricle refills with blood. This portion of the cardiac cycle is called the diastole. The outlet valve is closed during diastole because the arterial pressure is greater than the intraventricular pressure. After the period of diastolic filling, the systolic phase of a new cardiac cycle is initiated.

6.2.2 Basic Requirements for Effective Ventricular Pumping

In order for the heart to perform effective ventricular pumping, the heart must operate normally in five basic ways: 1) the contraction of individual myocardial cells must occur periodically and synchronously; 2) the valve must be fully open without narrowing; 3) the valve must be completely closed without leakage or backflow; 4) muscle contractions must be strong; 5) the ventricles must be fully filled during the diastole.

Some investigators demonstrated that as cardiac filling increases during diastole, the volume ejected during systole also increases. As a consequence with other factors equal, stroke volume increases as the cardiac end-diastolic volume increases. This phenomenon (commonly referred to as the law of the heart) is an intrinsic property of the cardiac muscle and is one of the primary regulators of cardiac output.

6.2.3 Autonomic Neural Influences

While the heart can inherently beat on its own, cardiac function can be influenced profoundly by neural inputs from both the sympathetic nerves and parasympathetic nerves divisions of the autonomic nervous system. These inputs allow us to modify cardiac pumping as is appropriate to meet changing homeostatic needs of the body. All portions of the heart are richly innervated by adrenergic sympathetic fibers. When active, these sympathetic nerves release norepinephrine on cardiac cells. Norepinephrine interacts with β_1-adrenergic receptors on cardiac muscle cells to increase heart rate, increase action potential conduction velocity, and increase force of contraction and rates of contraction and relaxation. Overall, sympathetic action acts to increase cardiac pumping.

Cholinergic parasympathetic fibers travel to the heart via the vagus nerve and innervate the sinoatrial node, the atrioventricular node, and the atrial muscle (心房肌). When active, these parasympathetic nerves release acetylcholine on cardiac muscle cells. Acetylcholine interacts with muscarinic receptors on cardiac muscle cells to decrease heart rate (SA node), decrease action potential conduction velocity (AV node). Parasympathetic nerves may also act to decrease the force of contraction of the atrial (not ventricular) muscle cells. Overall, parasympathetic activation acts to decrease cardiac pumping. Usually an increase in parasympathetic nerve activity is accompanied by a decrease in sympathetic nerve activity, and vice versa.

6.3　Vasculature

Blood that is ejected into the aorta by the left heart passes consecutively through many different types of vessels before it returns to the right heart. The major vessel classifications are arteries, arterioles, capillaries, venules and veins. These consecutive vascular segments are distinguished from one another by differences in physical dimensions, morphological characteristics, and function. One feature that all vessels have in common is that they are lined with a contiguous single layer of endothelial cells. In fact, this is true for the entire circulatory system including the heart chambers and even the valve leaflets.

Arteries are thick-walled vessels that contain, in addition to some smooth muscle, a large component of elastin and collagen fibers. Primarily because of the elastin fibers, which can stretch to twice their unloaded length, arteries can expand to accept and temporarily store some of the blood ejected by the heart during systole. The aorta is the largest artery and has an inside diameter of about 25mm. Arterial diameter decreases with each consecutive branching. The smallest arteries have diameters of approximately 0.1mm.

Arterioles are smaller and structured differently than arteries. In proportion to lumen size, arterioles have much thicker walls with more smooth muscle and less elastic material than arteries. Because arterioles are so muscular, their diameters can be actively changed to regulate the blood flow through peripheral organs. Arterioles are often referred to as the resistance vessels because of their high and changeable resistance, which regulates peripheral blood flow through individual organs. Capillaries are the smallest vessels in the vasculature. The capillary wall consists of a single layer of endothelial cells, which separate the blood from the interstitial fluid by only a few micrometers. Capillaries contain no smooth muscle and thus lack the ability to change their diameters actively. For obvious reasons, capillaries are viewed as the exchange vessels of the cardiovascular system. In addition to the diffusion of solutes that occurs across these vessel walls, there can sometimes be net move-

ments of fluid into and/or out of capillaries. For example, edema is a result of net fluid movement from plasma into the interstitial space.

After leaving capillaries, blood is collected in venules and veins and then returned to the heart. Venous vessels have very thin walls in proportion to their diameters. Their walls contain smooth muscle and the diameters of venous vessels can actively change. Because of their thin walls, venous vessels are quite distensible. Therefore, their diameters change passively in response to small changes in transmural distending pressure. Venous vessels, especially the larger ones, also have one-way valves that prevent reverse flow. As it will be discussed later, these valves are especially important in the cardiovascular system's operation during standing and during exercise. It turns out that peripheral venules and veins normally contain more than 50% of the total blood volume. Consequently, they are commonly thought of as the capacitance vessels. More importantly changes in venous volume greatly influence cardiac filling and therefore cardiac pumping. Thus, peripheral veins actually play an extremely important role in controlling cardiac output.

Blood flow through individual vascular beds is profoundly influenced by changes in activity of sympathetic nerves innervating arterioles. These nerves release norepinephrine from their endings which interacts with α-adrenergic receptors on the smooth muscle cells to cause contraction and thus arteriolar constriction. The reduction in arteriolar diameter increases vascular resistance and decreases blood flow. These neural fibers provide the most important means of reflex control over vascular resistance and organ blood flow.

Arteriolar smooth muscle is also very responsive to changes in the local chemical conditions within an organ that accompany changes in the metabolic rate of the organ. For reasons to be discussed later, an increased tissue metabolic rate leads to arteriolar dilation and an increased tissue blood flow.

Venules and veins are also richly innervated by sympathetic nerves and constrict when these nerves are activated. The mechanism is the same as that involved with arterioles. Thus, increased sympathetic nerve activity is accompanied by decreased venous volume. The importance of this phenomenon is that venous constriction tends to increase cardiac filling and, therefore, cardiac output via Starling's law of the heart.

There is no important neural or local metabolic control of either the arterial or capillary vessels.

Summary

心脏是推动血液流动的动力器官，其主要功能是泵血。心脏泵血主要由两个因素决定：一是心脏节律性收缩和舒张建立的心室、心房与动静脉之间的压力梯度，二是心脏瓣膜的单向开启和闭合控制血流方向。机体能够通过改变心室的充盈和支配心脏的自主神经活动来改变心输出量以适应机体的功能活动。同时机体能够通过改变交感神经活动和局部环境的物质来改变小动脉直径，进而调节各器官中的血流量。

Xiao Yu (肖宇)

Chapter 7　Characteristics of Cardiac Muscle Cells

7.1　Electrical Activity of Cardiac Muscle Cells

Cardiac muscle cell action potentials differ sharply from those of skeletal muscle cells in three important ways that promote synchronous rhythmic excitation of the heart: 1) they can be self-generating; 2) they can be conducted directly from cell to cell; 3) they have long durations, which preclude fusion of individual twitch contractions.

7.1.1　Resting Potential

All cells have an electrical potential across their membranes. Such membrane potential exists because the ions concentration in the cytoplasm are different from those of the interstitium and ions diffusing down concentration gradients across semipermeable membranes generates electrical gradients. The three ions that are the most important determinants of cardiac membrane potential are sodium ions and calcium ions and potassium ions. With the normal concentrations of about 145mmol/L K^+ inside cells and mmol/L K^+ in the extracellular fluid, the potassium equilibrium potential is roughly –90mV (more negative inside than outside by 90mV). A membrane that is permeable only to K^+ will inherently and rapidly develop the potassium equilibrium potential. Under resting conditions, most heart muscle cells have membrane potentials that are quite close to the potassium equilibrium potential.

7.1.2　Cardiac Cell Action Potentials

Fast response action potentials (Fig. 7-1) are characterized by a rapid depolarization period (phase 0) with a substantial overshoot, a rapid early repolarization (phase 1) of the overshoot potential, a plateau (phase 2), and an end of rapid repolarization (phase 3) to a stable resting period (phase 4).

In comparison, the slow response action potentials are characterized by a slower initial depolarization

phase, a lower amplitude overshoot, a shorter and less stable plateau, and repolarization to an unstable, slowly depolarizing resting potential. The unstable resting potential seen in pacemaker cells with slow response action potentials is variously referred to as the phase 4 automatic depolarization, diastolic depolarization, or pacemaker potential.

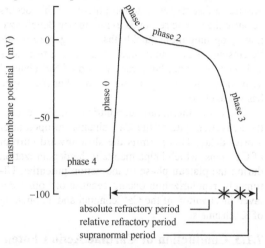

Figure 7-1　Cardiac cell action potentials.

Firstly, there is a progressive decrease in the membrane's permeability to K^+ during the resting phase, and secondly, the permeability to Na^+ increases slightly. The gradual increase in the Na^+/K^+ permeability ratio will cause the membrane potential to move slowly away from the K^+ equilibrium potential (–90mV) towards the direction of the Na^+ equilibrium potential. Lastly, there is an increase in the permeability of the membrane to calcium ions, which results in an inward movement of positively charged ions and also contributes to the diastolic depolarization.

When the membrane potential depolarizes to a certain threshold potential in either type of cell, major rapid alterations in the permeability changes cannot be stopped until they proceed to completion.

The characteristic rapid rising phase of the fast response action potential is a result of a sudden increase in Na^+ permeability. This produces what is referred to as fast inward current of Na^+ and causes the membrane potential to move rapidly toward the sodium equilibrium potential. This period of very high sodium permeability is short-lived. It is followed by a more slowly developed increase in the membrane's permeability to Ca^{2+} and a decrease in its permeability to K^+.

Cells are in an **absolute refractory period** (绝对不应期) during most of the action potential (they cannot be stimulated to fire another action potential). Near the end of the action potential, the membrane is in **relative refractory period** (相对不应期) and can be excited only by a larger than normal stimulus. Immediately after the action potential, the membrane is transiently hyperexcitable and is said to be in a **supranormal period** (超常期).

In the resting state, with the membrane polarized to near $-80mV$, the activation or m gate of the fast Na^+ channel is closed, but its inactivation or h gate is open. With a rapid depolarization of the membrane to threshold potential, the Na^+ channels will be activated strongly to allow an inrush of positive sodium ions that further depolarizes the membrane and thus initiates a fast response action potential. This occurs because the m gate responds to membrane depolarization by opening more quickly than the h gate responds by closing. Thus a rapid depolarization to threshold is followed by a brief but strong period of Na^+ channel activation wherein the m gate is open but the h gate has yet to close.

The initial membrane depolarization also causes the activation gate of the Ca^{2+} channel to open after a brief delay. This permits the slow inward current of Ca^{2+} ions, which helps maintain the depolarization during the plateau phase of the action potential. Ultimately, repolarization occurs because of both a delayed inactivation of the Ca^{2+} channel and an opening of K^+ channels.

7.1.3 Conduction of Cardiac Action Potentials

Action potentials are conducted over the surface of individual cells because active depolarization in any one area of the membrane produces local currents in the intracellular and extracellular fluid which passively depolarize immediately adjacent areas of the membrane to their voltage threshold for active depolarization.

In the heart, cardiac muscle cells are connected end-to-end by structures called intercalated disks. These intercalated disks contain the following: 1) firm mechanical attachments between adjacent cell membranes by proteins called adhesins in structures called demosomes; 2) low resistance electrical connections between adjacent cells through channels formed by protein called connexin, in structures called gap junctions. Thus, an action potential initiated at any site in the myocardium will be conducted cell-to-cell throughout the entire myocardium.

The speed at which an action potential propagates through a region of cardiac tissue is called the conduction velocity. The conduction velocity varies considerably in different areas in the heart. This velocity is directly dependent on the diameter of the muscle fiber involved. Thus, conduction over small diameter cells in the AV node is significantly slower than conduction over large-diameter cells in the ventricular

Purkinje system. Conduction velocity is also directly dependent on the intensity of the local depolarization currents, which are in turn directly determined by the rate of rise of the action potential. Rapid depolarization favors rapid conduction. Variations in the capacitive and/or resistive properties of the cell membranes, gap junctions, and cytoplasm are also factors that contribute to the differences in conduction velocity of action potentials through specific areas of the heart.

Specific electrical adaptations of various cells in the heart are reflected in the characteristic shape of their action potentials. Cells of the sinoatrial node serve as the heart's normal **pacemaker** (起搏点) and determine the heart rate. This is because the **spontaneous depolarization** (自动去极化) of the resting membrane is most rapid in sinoatrial node cells. The action potential initiated by sinoatrial node cells first spreads progressively through the atrial wall.

Action potential conduction is greatly slowed as it passes through the artrioventricular node. This is because of the small size of the artrioventricular node cells and the slow rate of rise of their action potentials. Since the AV node delays the transfer of the cardiac excitation from the atria to the ventricles, the ventricles contraction can occur just after atrial contraction.

Because of sharply rising action potentials and other factors, such as large cell diameters, electrical conduction is extremely rapid in Purkinje fibers. This allows the Purkinje system to transfer the cardiac impulse to cells in many areas of the ventricle nearly in unison.

7.1.4 Effect of Heart Rate

Normal rhythmic contractions of the heart occur because of spontaneous electrical pacemaker activity (automaticity) of cells in the sinoatrial node. The heart rate is determined by how long it takes the membranes of these pacemaker cells to spontaneously depolarize to the threshold level. The SA node cells fire at a spontaneous or intrinsic rate (approximately equal to 100 beats per minute) in the absence of any outside influences.

The two most important outside influences on the automaticity of SA node cells come from the autonomic nervous system. Fibers from both the sympathetic and parasympathetic divisions of the autonomic system terminate on cells in the SA node, and these fibers can modify the intrinsic heart rate. Activating the cardiac sympathetic nerves increases the heart rate. Increasing cardiac parasympathetic tone slows the heart rate. The parasympathetic and sympathetic nerves both influence the heart rate by altering the course of spontaneous depolarization of the resting potential in SA pacemaker cells.

Cardiac parasympathetic fibers, which travel to the heart through the vagus nerves, release the neurotransmitter substance acetylcholine onto SA node cells. Acetylcholine increases the permeability of the resting membrane to K^+. These permeability changes have two effects on the resting potential of cardiac pacemaker cells: 1) They cause an initial hyperpolarization of the resting membrane potential by bringing it closer to the K^+ equilibrium potential. 2) They slow the rate of spontaneous depolarization of the resting membrane. Both of these effects increase the time between beats by prolonging the time required for the resting membrane to depolarize to the threshold level. Since there are normally some continuous nerve impulses of cardiac parasympathetic nerves, the normal resting heart rate is approximately 70 beats per minute.

Sympathetic nerves release the neurotransmitter substance norepinephrine onto cardiac cells. Norepinephrine increases the inward currents carried by Na^+ and by Ca^{2+}. These changes will increase the heart rate by accelerating the rate of diastolic depolarization.

In addition to sympathetic and parasympathetic nerves, there are many factors that can alter the heart rate. These factors include a number of ions and circulating hormones, as well as physical influences such as temperature and atrial wall stretch. All act by somehow altering the time required for the resting membrane to depolarize to the threshold potential. An abnormally high concentration of Ca^{2+} in the extracellular fluid, for example, tends to decrease the heart rate by shifting the threshold potential. Factors that increase the heart rate are said to have a positive chronotropic action. Those that decrease the heart rate have a negative chronotropic action.

Besides their effect on the heart rate, autonomic fibers also influence the conduction velocity of action potentials through the heart. Increase in sympathetic activity increases conduction velocity having a positive dromotropic action, whereas increase in parasympathetic activity decreases conduction velocity having a negative dromotropic action. These effects are most notable at the SA node and can influence the duration of the P-R interval.

7.2　Cardiac Muscle Contraction

Contraction of the myocardial cell is initiated by the action potential. Contraction evokes tension generation and/or shortening of the cell.

7.2.1　Excitation-contraction Coupling

Muscle action potential triggers mechanical contraction through a process called excitation-contraction coupling. The major event in excitation-contraction coupling is a dramatic rise in the intracellular free Ca^{2+} concentration. The resting state intracellular free Ca^{2+} concentration is less than $0.1 \mu mol/L$. In contrast, during maximum activation of the contractile apparatus, the intracellular free Ca^{2+} concentration reaches nearly $100 \mu mol/L$. When the wave of depolarization

passes over the muscle cell membrane and down the T tubules, Ca^{2+} is released from the sarcoplasmic reticulum into the intracellular fluid.

The specific trigger for this release appears to be the entry of calcium into the cell via the L-type calcium channels and an increase in Ca^{2+} concentration in the region just under the sarcolemma on the surface of the cell and throughout the T-tubular system. Unlike skeletal muscle, this highly localized increase in calcium is essential for triggering the massive release of calcium from the sarcoplasmic reticulum (肌质网, SR). This calcium-induced calcium release is a result of opening calcium-sensitive release channels on the SR. Although the amount of Ca^{2+} that enters the cell during a single action potential is quite small compared with that released from the SR, it is not only essential for triggering the SR calcium release but also essential for maintaining adequate levels of Ca^{2+} in the intracellular stores over the long run.

When the intracellular Ca^{2+} level is high ($>0.1 \mu mol/L$), links called cross-bridges form between the two types of filaments found within muscle. Sarcomere units are joined end to end at Z lines to form myofibrils, which determine the length of the muscle cell. During contraction, thick and thin filaments slide past one another to shorten each sarcomere and thus the muscle. The bridges form when the regularly spaced myosin heads from thick filaments attach to regularly spaced sites on the action molecules in the thin filaments. Subsequent deformation of the bridges result in a pulling of the actin molecules toward the center of the sarcomere. This actin-myosin interaction requires energy from ATP. In resting muscles, the attachment of myosin to the actin sites is inhibited by troponin and tropomyosin. Calcium causes muscle contraction by interacting with troponin C to cause a configurational change that removes the inhibition of the actin sites on the thin filament. Since a single cross-bridge is a very short structure, gross muscle shortening requires that cross-bridges repetitively form, produce incremental movement between the myofilaments, detach, form again at a new actin site, and so on, in a cyclic manner.

There are several processes that participate in the reduction of intracellular Ca^{2+} that terminate the contraction. Approximately 80% of the calcium is actively taken back into the SR by the action of Ca^{2+}-ATPase pumps located in the network part of the SR. About 20% of the calcium is extruded from the cell into the extracellular fluid either via the Na^+-Ca^{2+} exchanger located in the sarcolemma or via Ca^{2+}-ATPase pumps of sarcolemma.

The duration of the cardiac muscle cell contraction is approximately the same as that of its action potential. Therefore, the electrical refractory period of a cardiac cell is not over until the mechanical response is completed. As a consequence, heart muscle cells cannot be activated rapidly enough to use a fused (tetanic) state of prolonged contraction. This is fortunate because intermittent contraction and relaxation are essential for the heart's pumping action.

7.2.2 Isometric Contractions

The active tension developed by cardiac muscle during the course of an isometric contraction depends very much on the muscle length at which the contraction occurs. Active tension development is maximal at some intermediate length referred to as L_{max}. Little active tension is developed at very short or very long muscle lengths. Histological studies indicate that the changes in the resting length of the whole muscle are associated with proportional changes in the individual sarcomeres. Peak tension development occurs at sarcomere lengths of 2.2 to 2.3μm. At sarcomere lengths shorter than 2.0μm, the opposing thin filaments may overlap or buckle, and thus interfering with active tension development.

7.2.3 Isotonic Contraction

During what is termed isotonic contraction, a muscle shortens against a constant load. Muscles exhibit isotonic contractions when lifting a fixed weight. Because **the preload** (前负荷) determines the resting muscle length, the factors that affect the extent of cardiac muscle shortening during an **afterload** (后负荷) contraction are of special interest to us.

7.2.4 Myocardial Contractility

A number of factors in addition to **initial length of muscle** (肌肉初长度) can affect the tension-generating potential of cardiac muscle. Any intervention which can increase the maximal tension at a fixed **initial length of muscle** is believed to increase myocardial contractility. Such an agent is said to have a positive inotropic action on the heart.

The most important physiological regulator of myocardial contractility is norepinephrine. When norepinephrine is released on cardiac muscle cells from sympathetic nerves; it has not only the chronotropic action on the heart rate as discussed earlier but also a pronounced positive inotropic action that causes cardiac muscle cells to contract more rapidly and forcefully.

Norepinephrine raises the peak isometric tension curve on the cardiac muscle length-tension curve. Norepinephrine is believed to increase myocardial contractility because it enhances the forcefulness of muscle contraction even when the length is constant. Changes in contractility and initial length can occur simultaneously, but by definition a change in contractility must involve a shift from one peak isometric length-tension curve to another.

The cellular mechanism of the norepinephrine effect on contractility is mediated by its interaction with a β_1-adrenergic receptor. The signaling pathway involves an activation of the Gs protein-cAMP-protein kinase A, which then phosphorylates the Ca^{2+} channel increasing the inward calcium current during plateau phase of the action potential. This increase in calcium influx not only contributes to the magnitude of the rise in intracellular Ca^{2+} for a given beat but also loads the internal calcium stores, which allows more to be released during subsequent depolarizations. This increase in free Ca^{2+} during activation allows more cross-bridges to be formed and greater tension to be developed.

Because norepinephrine also causes phosphorylation of the regulatory protein on the sarcoplasmic reticular Ca^{2+} ATPase pump, the rate of calcium getting back into the SR is enhanced and the rate of relaxation is increased. This is called a positive lusitropic action. In addition to accelerating SR calcium recovery, norepinephrine also results in a decrease in action potential duration. This effect is achieved by a potassium channel alteration, occurring in response to the elevated intracellular $[Ca^{2+}]$. That increases potassium permeability, terminates the plateau of the action potential and contributes to the early relaxation. Such shortening of the systolic interval is helpful in the presence of elevated heart rates, that might otherwise significantly compromise diastolic filling time.

Enhanced parasympathetic activity has been shown to have a small negative inotropic action upon the heart. In the atria, where this action is most pronounced, the negative inotropic action is thought to be due to a shortening of the action potential and a decrease in the amount of Ca^{2+} that enters the cell during the action potential.

Summary

心脏实现其泵血功能是以心肌的收缩和舒张为基础的，但心房和心室之所以能不停地进行有顺序的、协调的收缩与舒张交替的活动，归根结底都是由心肌细胞动作电位的规律性发生与扩布而引起的。正常起搏点窦房结P细胞动作电位3期复极化末在达到最大复极电位后，4期的膜电位并不稳定于这一水平，而是立即开始自动去极化，当去极化达阈电位水平时，即爆发一次新的动作电位。窦房结的自律性最高，由它发出的节律性兴奋依次激动心房肌、房室交界、房室束、心室内传导组织和心室肌，心室肌细胞发生跨膜电位，通过兴奋收缩偶联，引起整个心脏的节律性兴奋和收缩。心室肌细胞在兴奋后也会发生兴奋性的周期性的变化即绝对不应期、相对不应期和超常期，由于心室肌细胞的绝对不应期特别长，所以，心肌细胞不会发生强直性收缩。无论是心脏的电生理特性还是其机械收缩特性，均受自主神经即交感神经和副交感神经的调控。自主神经对于心肌细胞的传导性，收缩性和自律性均有明显的影响。

Xiao Yu (肖宇)

Chapter 8　Pump Function

8.1　Cardiac Cycle

A **cardiac cycle** (心动周期) is defined as one complete sequence of ventricular contraction and relaxation.

8.1.1　Ventricular Diastole

The **diastolic period** (舒张期) of the cardiac cycle begins with the opening of the atrioventricular valves. The mitral valve opens when the left ventricular pressure falls below the left atrial pressure and the period of ventricle filling begins. Blood that had previously accumulated in the atrium behind the closed mitral valve empties rapidly into the ventricle and this causes an initial drop in the atrial pressure. Later, the pressures in both chambers slowly rise together as the atrium and ventricle continue passively filling in unison with blood returning to the heart through the veins.

Atrial contraction is initiated near the end of ventricular diastole by the depolarization of the atrial muscle cells, which causes the P wave of the electrocardiogram. As the atrial muscle cells develop tension and shorten, the atrial pressure rises and an additional amount of blood is forced into the ventricle. At normal heart rates, atrial contraction is not essential for adequate ventricular filling. After atrial contraction, the ventricle nearly reaches to its maximum volume, and the ventricular volume at this point is known as **end-diastolic volume** (EDV, 舒张末期容积).

8.1.2　Ventricular Systole

Ventricular systole begins when the action potential breaks through the atrioventricular node and spreads all over the ventricular muscles, an event heralded by the QRS complex of the electrocardiogram. Contraction of the ventricular muscle cells causes intraventricular pressure to rise above that in the atrium, which causes abrupt closure of the AV valve.

Pressure in the left ventricle continues to rise sharply as the ventricular contraction intensifies. When the left ventricular pressure exceeds that in the aorta, the aortic valve opens. The period of time between mitral valve closure and aortic valve opening is referred to as the **isovolumic contraction phase** (等容收缩期) because during this interval the ventricle is a closed chamber with a fixed volume. Ventricular ejection begins with the opening of the aortic valve. In early ejection phase, blood enters the aorta rapidly and causes the pressure there to rise. Pressure builds simultaneously in both the ventricle and the aorta as the ventricular muscle cells continue to contract in early systole. This period is often called the **rapid ejection phase** (快速射血期).

Left ventricular and aortic pressures ultimately reach their maximum called **the systolic pressure** (SP, 收缩压). At this point the strength of ventricular muscle contraction begins to wane. Muscle shortening and ejection continue, but at a reduced rate. Aortic pressure begins to fall because blood is leaving the aorta and large arteries faster than blood is entering from the left ventricle. Throughout ejection, very small pressure differences exist between the left ventricle and the aorta because the valve orifice is so large that it presents very little resistance to flow.

Eventually, the strength of the ventricular contraction diminishes to the point where the intraventricular pressure falls below the aortic pressure. This causes abrupt closure of the aortic valve. After aortic valve closure, the intraventricular pressure falls rapidly as the ventricular muscle relaxes. For a brief interval, called the **isovolumetric relaxation phase** (等容舒张期), the mitral valve is also closed. Ultimately, the intraventricular pressure falls below the atrial pressure, the AV valve opens, and a new cardiac cycle begins.

The amount of blood ejected from the ventricle during a single beat, the stroke volume is equal to end-diastolic volume minus end-systolic volume.

The aorta distends or balloons out during systole because more blood enters the aorta than leaving it. During diastole, the arterial pressure is maintained by the elastic recoil of the walls of the aorta and other large arteries. Nonetheless, aortic pressure gradually falls during diastole as the aorta supplies blood to the systemic vascular beds. The lowest aortic pressure, reached at the end of diastole, is called the **diastolic** pressure (舒张压). The difference between the diastolic and peak systolic pressure in the aorta is called the arterial **pulse pressure** (脉压). Typical values for systolic and diastolic pressures in the aorta are 120 and 80mmHg, respectively.

At a normal resting heart rate of about 70 beats per minute, the heart spends approximately two-thirds of the cardiac cycle in diastole and one-third in systole. When increase in the heart rate occurs, both diastolic and systolic intervals become shorter. Action potential durations are shortened and conduction velocity is increased. Contraction and relaxation rates are also enhanced. This shortening of the systolic interval tends to blunt the potential adverse effects of an increased heart rate on diastolic filling time.

8.2　Heart Sounds

A **phonocardiogram** (心音图) records the heart sounds, which occur during the cardiac cycle. **The first heart sound** (S_1, 第一心音) occurs at the beginning of systole because of the abrupt closure of the artrioventricular valves, which produces vibrations of the cardiac structures and the blood in the ventricular chambers. S_1 can be heard most clearly by placing the stethoscope over the apex of the heart. Note that this sound occurs immediately after the QRS complex of **the electrocardiogram** (ECG, 心电图).

The second heart sound (S_2, 第二心音), arises from the closure of the aortic and pulmonary valves at the beginning of the period of isovolumetric relaxation. This sound is heard around the time of the T wave on the electrocardiogram. The pulmonary valve usually closes slightly after the aortic valve.

The third heart sound (S_3, 第三心音) and **the fourth heart sound** (S_4, 第四心音) are not normally present. When they are present, however, they along with S_1 and S_2, produce what are called the gallop rhythm. When present, the third heart sound occurs shortly after S_2 during the period of rapid passive ventricular filling and, in combination with heart sounds S_1 and S_2, produces what is called the ventricular gallop rhythm. Although S_3 may sometimes be detected in normal children, it is heard more commonly in patients with left ventricular failure. The fourth heart sound, which occasionally is heard shortly before S_1, is associated with the atrial contraction and rapid active filling of the ventricle.

8.3　Measurement of Cardiac Function

8.3.1　Cardiac Output & Cardiac Index

Cardiac output: It is referred to liters of blood pumped by each of the ventricles per minute. The normal cardiac output for an individual is obviously dependent on his or her size. For example, the cardiac output of a 50kg woman will be significantly lower than that of a 90kg man. It has been found, however, that cardiac output correlates better with body surface area than with body weight. Therefore, it is common to express the cardiac output per square meter of surface area. This value is called **the cardiac index** (心指数) and at rest, it is normally approximately $3L/(min \cdot m^2)$.

8.3.2　Stroke Volume & Ejection Fraction

The volume of blood emitted from one ventricle in one heart stroke is called the stroke volume. Stroke volume is equal to ventricular end-diastolic volume minus ventricular end-systolic volume.

Ejection fraction (EF, 射血分数) is an extremely useful clinical measurement. It is defined as the ratio of stroke volume to end-diastolic volume: $EF = SV/EDV$. Ejection fraction is commonly expressed as a percentage and normally ranges from 55% to 65% under testing conditions. Ejection fractions of less than 55% indicate depressed myocardial contractility.

8.4　Determinants of Cardiac Output

Cardiac output (liters of blood pumped by each of the ventricles per minute) is an extremely important cardiovascular variable that is continuously adjusted so that the cardiovascular system operates to meet the body's moment-to-moment transport needs. In going from rest to strenuous exercise, for example, the cardiac output of an average person will increase from approximately 5.0 to perhaps 30L/min.

Cardiac output is the product of heart rate and stroke volume ($CO = HR \times SV$). Therefore, all changes in cardiac output must be produced by changes in heart rate and/or stroke volume.

Factors influencing heart rate do so by altering the characteristics of the diastolic depolarization of the pacemaker cells. Recall that variations in activity of the sympathetic and parasympathetic nerves leading to cells of the SA node constitute the most important regulators of heart rate. Increase in sympathetic activity increases heart rate whereas increase in parasympathetic activity decreases heart rate. These neural inputs have immediate effects (within one beat) and therefore can cause very rapid adjustments in cardiac output.

Heart rate is controlled by chronotropic actions on the spontaneous electrical activity of SA node cells. Cardiac parasympathetic nerves have a negative chronotropic action, and sympathetic nerves have a positive chronotropic action on the SA node. Stroke volume is controlled by influences on the contractile performance of ventricular cardiac muscle in particular its degree of shortening in the afterload situation. The three distinct influences on stroke volume are myocardial contractility, preload, and afterload. Increased cardiac sympathetic nerve activity tends to increase stroke volume by increasing the myocardial contractility. Increased arterial pressure tends to decrease stroke volume by increasing the afterload on cardiac muscle fibers. Increased ventricular filling pressure increases end-diastolic volume, which tends to increase stroke volume through Starling's law.

8.5 Influences on Stroke Volume

8.5.1 Effect of Changes in Ventricular Preload: Frank-Starling Law

The volume of blood that the heart ejects with each heartbeat can vary significantly. One of the most important factors responsible for these variations in stroke volume is the extent of cardiac filling during diastole. This law states that, with other factors equal, stroke volume increases as cardiac filling increases. As we will now show, this phenomenon is based on the intrinsic mechanical properties of myocardial cells.

Recall from the nature of the resting length-tension relationship that an increased preload is necessarily accompanied by increased initial muscle fiber length. When a muscle starts from a greater length, it has more room to shorten before it reaches the length at which its tension-generating capability is no longer greater than the load upon it. The same behavior is exhibited by cardiac muscle cells when they are actually operating in the ventricular wall. An increase in ventricular preload results in an increase in both end-diastolic volume and stroke volume, almost equally. The precise relationship between cardiac preload (cardiac filling pressure) and end-diastolic volume has especially important physiological and clinical consequences.

Increasing preload increases initial muscle length without significantly changing the final length to which the muscle shortens against a constant total load. Thus, increasing ventricular filling pressure increases stroke volume primarily by increasing end-diastolic volume. This is not accompanied by a significant alteration in end-systolic volume.

8.5.2 Effect of Changes in Ventricular Afterload

As stated previously, systemic arterial pressure (ventricular afterload) is analogous to total load in isolated muscle experiments. A slight complication is that arterial pressure varies between diastolic value and systolic value during each cardiac ejection. Usually, however, we are interested in mean ventricular afterload and take this to be **mean arterial pressure** (平均动脉压).

Increased afterload, at constant preload, has a neg-

ative impact on cardiac muscle shortening. Again, this is simply a consequence of the fact that muscle cannot shorten beyond the length at which its peak isometric tension-generating potential equals the total load upon it. Thus, shortening must stop at a greater muscle length when afterload is increased. In a normally functioning heart, the effect of changes in afterload on end-systolic volume (and therefore stroke volume) is quite small (about 0.5mL/mmHg). However, in what is termed systolic cardiac failure the effect of afterload on end-systolic volume is greatly enhanced. Thus, the slope of this line can be used clinically to assess the systolic function of the heart.

8.5.3 Effect of Changes in Myocardial Contractility

Recall that activation of the sympathetic nervous system results in release of norepinephrine from cardiac sympathetic nerves which increases contractility of the individual cardiac muscle cells. This results in an upward shift of the peak isometric length-tension curve. Such a shift will result in an increase in the shortening of a muscle contracting with constant preload and total load. Thus, the norepinephrine released by sympathetic nerve stimulation will increase ventricular stroke volume by decreasing the end-systolic volume without directly influencing the end-diastolic volume.

8.6 Cardiac Function Curves

One very useful way to summarize the influences on cardiac function and the interactions between them is by cardiac function curves, such as those shown in Fig. 8-1. In this case, cardiac output is treated as the dependent variable and is plotted on the vertical axis in Fig. 8-1, while cardiac filling pressure is plotted on the horizontal axis.

Different curves are used to show the influence of alterations in sympathetic nerve activity. Thus, Fig. 8-1 shows how the cardiac filling pressure and the activity level of cardiac sympathetic nerves interact to determine cardiac output. When cardiac filling pressure is 2mmHg and the activity of cardiac sympathetic nerves is normal, the heart will operate at point A and will have a cardiac output of 5L/min. Each single curve in Fig. 8-1 shows how cardiac output would be changed by changes in cardiac filling pressure if cardiac sympathetic nerve activity were held at a fixed level. For example, if cardiac sympathetic nerve activity remained normal, increasing cardiac filling pressure from 2 to 4mmHg would cause the heart to shift its operation from point A to point B on the cardiac function diagram. In this case, cardiac output would increase from 5 to 7mL/min solely as a result of the increased filling pressure (Starling's law). If, on the other hand, cardiac filling pressure is fixed

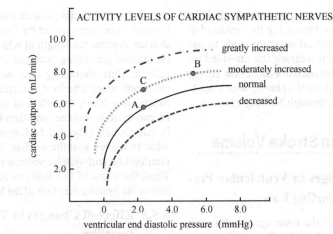

Figure 8-1 Influence of cardiac sympathetic nerves on cardiac function curves.

at 2mmHg while the activity of cardiac sympathetic nerves is moderately increased from normal, the heart would change from operating at point A to operating at point C. Cardiac output would again increase from 5 to 7mL/min. In this instance, however, cardiac output does not increase through the length-dependent mechanism because cardiac filling pressure did not change. Cardiac output increases at constant filling pressure with an increase in cardiac sympathetic activity for two reasons. Firstly, increased cardiac sympathetic nerve activity increases heart rate. Secondly, but just as important, increased sympathetic nerve activity increases stroke volume by increasing myocardial contractility.

Summary

心脏泵血依靠心脏收缩和舒张的交替活动而得以完成。心脏的一次收缩和舒张，构成一个机械活动周期，称为心动周期。心室收缩期可分为等容收缩期和射血期，而射血期又可分为快速射血期和减慢射血期。心室舒张期可分为等容舒张期和心室充盈期，心室充盈期又可分为快速充盈期、减慢充盈期和心房收缩期。

在心动周期中，心肌收缩、瓣膜启闭、血液流速改变形成的涡流和血液撞击心室壁及大动脉壁引起的振动，可通过周围组织传递到胸壁，用听诊器便可在胸部某些部位听到，这就是心音。正常心脏在一次搏动过程中，可产生4个心音，即第一、第二、第三和第四心音。通常用听诊的方法只能听到第一和第二心音；在某些青年人和健康儿童可听到第三心音；用心音图可记录到4个心音。

在临床医学实践和科学工作中，常常需要对心脏的泵血功能进行判断，或对心脏的功能状态进行评价。对心脏泵血功能的评定，通常用单位时间内心脏的射血量即每搏输出量、射血分数、每分输出量和心指数进行评价。心输出量等于搏出量与心率的乘积，因此凡能影响搏出量和心率的因素均可影响心输出量。而搏出量的多少则决定于前负荷、后负荷和心肌收缩能力等。

Xiao Yu（肖宇）

Chapter 9   Electrocardiogram

Fields of electrical potential generated by the electrical activity of the heart extend through the body tissue and can be measured with electrodes placed on the body surface. If the measuring electrode is placed in a certain part of the body surface, the electrical changes that occur during the process of heart excitation can be guided and is recorded on a special paper. This is called electrocardiogram. ECG can reflect the bioelectrical changes in the process of generating, conducting, and excitatory recovery of the whole heart, but not directly related to the mechanical contractile activity of the heart. ECG provides a record of how the voltage between two points on the body surface changes over time as a result of the electrical events of the cardiac cycle. At any instant of the cardiac cycle, the electrocardiogram indicates the net electrical field, that is the summation of many weak electrical fields being produced by voltage changes occurring on individual cardiac cells at that instant. When a large number of cells are simultaneously depolarization or repolarization, large voltages are observed on the electrocardiogram. Since the electrical impulse spreads through the heart tissue in a stereotyped manner, the temporal pattern of voltage change recorded between two points on the body surface is also stereotyped and will repeat itself with each heart cycle.

The typical ECG waveform and its physiological significance. There are horizontal lines and vertical lines on the ECG recording paper, and the small squares with 1mm length and width are drawn. When recording the electrocardiogram, first adjusting the magnification of the instrument to make the input 1mV voltage signal, the drawing pen produces 10mm offset in the longitudinal direction, so that each small lattice on the longitudinal line is equivalent to the 0.1mV potential difference. The horizontal lattices represent time, and each small square is equivalent to 0.04s (that is, the paper speed is 25mm per second). Therefore, the potential values and the duration of the ECG waves can be measured on the recording paper Fig. 9-1.

The major features of an electrocardiogram are the P wave, the QRS complex and the T wave. The P wave corresponds to atrial depolarization, the QRS complex to ventricular depolarization, and the T wave to ventricular repolarization.

9.1   Basic Features of Electrocardiogram

The major features of the electrocardiogram are the P wave, the QRS complex, and the T wave that are caused in turn by atrial depolarization, ventricular depolarization, and ventricular repolarization, respectively. The period of time from the initiation of the P wave to the beginning of the QRS complex is designated as the **P-R interval** (P-R间期) and indicates the time it takes for an action potential to spread through the atria and the atrioventricular node. During the latter portion of the P-R interval, no voltages are detected on the body surface. This is because atrial muscle cells are depolarized and in the plateau of their action potentials, ventricular cells are still at rest, and the electrical field set up by the action potential progressing through the small artrionventricular node is not intense enough to be detected. The duration of the normal P-R interval ranges from 120 to 200ms. Shortly after the cardiac impulse spreads out of the artrionventricular node and into the rapidly conducting Purkinje fibers, all the ventricular muscle cells depolarize within a very short period of time and cause the QRS complex. The R wave is the largest event in the electrocardiogram because ventricular muscle cells are so numerous and they depolarize nearly in unison. The normal QRS complex lasts between 60 and 100ms. The repolarization of atrial cells is also occurring during the time period in which ventricular depolarization generates the QRS complex on the electrocardiogram. Atrial repolarization is not evident on the electrocardiogram because it is a poorly synchronized event in a relatively small mass of heart tissue and is completely overshadowed by the major electrical events occurring in the ventricles at this time.

The QRS complex is followed by the ST segment. Normally, no electrical potentials are measured on the body surface during the ST segment because no rapid changes in membrane potential are occurring in any of the cells of the heart. Atrial cells have already returned to the resting phase, whereas ventricular muscle cells are in the plateau phase of their action potentials. Myocardial infarction or myocardial ischemia, however, can produce elevations or depressions in the

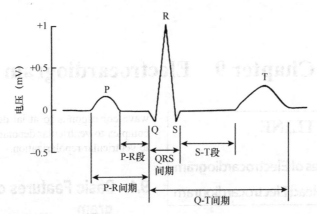

Figure 9-1 Electrocardiogram pattern.

ST segment. When ventricular cells begin to repolarize, a voltage once again appears on the body surface and is measured as the T wave of the electrocardiogram. The T wave is broader than and not as large as the R wave because ventricular repolarization is less synchronous than depolarization. At the conclusion of the T wave, all the cells in the heart are in the resting state. The Q-T interval roughly approximates the duration of the ventricular myocyte depolarization and thus the period of ventricular systole. At a normal heart rate of 60 beats/min, the Q-T interval is normally less than 380ms. No body surface potential is measured until the next impulse is generated by the sinoatrial node.

It should be recognized that the operation of the specialized conduction system is a primary factor in determining the normal electrocardiogram. For example, the artrionventricular node transmission time determines the P-R interval. Also, the effectiveness of the Purkinje system in synchronizing ventricular depolarization is reflected in the large magnitude and short duration of the QRS complex. It should also be noted that some heart muscle cells are inherently capable of automaticity, and many cardiac cells are electrically interconnected through gap junctions. Thus a functional heart rhythm can and often does occur without the involvement of part or all of the specialized conduction system. Such a situation is, however, abnormal, and the existence of abnormal conduction pathways would produce an abnormal electrocardiogram.

9.2 Standard 12-lead Electrocardiogram

The standard clinical electrocardiogram involves voltage measurements recorded from 12 different leads. Three of these are the bipolar limb leads Ⅰ, Ⅱ and Ⅲ. The other nine leads are unipolar limb leads. Three of these leads are generated using the limb electrodes. Two of the electrodes are electrically connected to form an indifferent electrode, while the third limb electrode is made the positive pole of the pair. Recordings made from these electrodes are called augmented unipolar limb leads. The voltage record obtained between the electrode at the right arm and the indifferent electrode is called a lead aVR electrocardiogram. Similarly lead aVL is recorded from the electrode on the left arm and lead aVF is recorded from the electrode on the left leg.

The standard limb leads (Ⅰ, Ⅱ and Ⅲ) and the augmented unipolar limb leads (aVR, aVL and aVF) record the electrical activity of the heart as it appears from six different perspectives, all in the frontal plane. The axes for leads Ⅰ, Ⅱ, and Ⅲ are those of the sides of Einthoven's triangle, while the axes for aVR, aVL and aVF are specified by lines drawn from the center of Einthoven's triangle to each of its vertices. The six limb leads can be thought of as a hexaxial reference system for observing the cardiac vectors in the frontal plane.

The other six leads of the standard 12-lead electrocardiogram are also unipolar leads that look at the electrical vector projections in the transverse plane. These potentials are obtained by placing an additional electrode in six specified positions on the chest wall. The indifferent electrode in this case is formed by electrically connecting the limb electrodes. These leads are identified as chest leads and are designated as V_1 to V_6. When the positive electrode is placed in position 1 and the wave of ventricular excitation sweeps away from it, the resultant deflection will be downward. When the electrode is in position 6 and the wave of ventricular excitation sweeps toward it, the deflection will be upward.

Summary

　　在正常人体，由窦房结发出的兴奋按一定的途径和时程依次传向心房和心室，引起整个心脏的兴奋。心脏各部分在兴奋过程中出现的生物电活动，可通过心脏周围的导电组织和体液传到体表。如果将测量电极置于体表的一定部位，即可引导出心脏兴奋过程中所发生的电变化，这种电变化经一定处理后并记录到特殊的记录纸上，便成为心电图。心电图可反映整个心脏兴奋的产生、传导和兴奋恢复过程中的生物电变化，而与心脏的机械收缩活动无直接关系。

正常典型心电图的波形及其生理意义：心电图记录纸上有横线和纵线划出长和宽均为1mm的小方格。记录心电图时，首先调节仪器放大倍数，使输入1mV电压信号时，描笔在纵向上产生10mm偏移，这样，纵线上每一小格相当于0.1mV

的电位差。横向小格表示时间，每一小格相当于0.04s（即走纸速度为每秒25mm）。因此，可以在记录纸上测量出心电图各波的电位数值和经历的时间。

心电图有多种导联，临床上检查心电图时，一般需要记录12个导联，包括Ⅰ、Ⅱ、Ⅲ三个标准导联，aVR、aVL、aVF三个加压单极肢体导联和$V_{1\sim6}$六个单极胸导联。主要以标准Ⅱ导联心电图为例，介绍心电图各波和间期的形态及其意义。

Wang Yuefei, Xiao Yu (王月飞，肖宇)

Chapter 10   Vascular Physiology

The vascular system connected with the heart is a relatively closed pipeline system. Through the flow of blood in the vessels, it realizes material transportation in the body and the important physiological functions such as tissue, cell material exchange and so on. All blood flows through the pulmonary circulation and the systemic circulation is made up of many parallel connected vascular circulation. In such a structure, even if the local blood flow is greatly changed, it will not have a great impact on the whole systemic circulation.

The vascular system of the systemic circulation and the pulmonary circulation is composed of the arteries, capillaries and veins. The arteries, the capillaries and the veins are connected in series, and both the systemic circulation and the pulmonary circulation are connected by the heart.

10.1 Classification of Blood Vessels

Blood vessels can be divided into the following categories from the physiological function: windkessel vessel, distributive vessel, precapillary resistance vessel, precapillary sphincter, exchange vessel, postcapillary resistance vessel, capacitance vessel and shunt vessel.

10.1.1 Windkessel Vessel

The main branch of the aorta and pulmonary artery and its largest branch, whose vascular wall is thick and rich in elastic fiber. It has obvious expansibility and elasticity, so it is called windkessel vessel.

10.1.2 Distribution Vessel

The function of the artery between the windkessel vessel and the arteriole is to transport the blood to the organs, so it is called distribution vessel.

10.1.3 Precapillary Resistance Vessel

Arterioles have small diameters and offer large resistance to blood flow, so they are called precapillary resistance vessels. The vascular walls of the arteriole are rich in smooth muscle, and their vasoconstriction can make the blood vessel diameter change obviously, so the blood flow resistance and the blood flow of the organ and tissue are changed.

10.1.4 Precapillary Sphincter

The beginning of the true capillaries is usually surrounded by smooth muscle, known as the precapillary sphincter. It can control the opening and closing of capillaries so that a number of capillaries can be opened and closed at any given time.

10.1.5 Exchange Vessel

The wall of the true capillaries is composed of a single layer of endothelial cells. There is a thin basement membrane outside. The true capillary permeability is very high. The real capillaries become the place for substance exchange between plasma and interstitial fluid, so they are called exchange vessel.

10.1.6 Postcapillary Resistance Vessel

Because of its small diameter, the venule also has some resistance to blood flow, so it is called postcapillary resistance vessel. The contractile and diastolic functions of the venule can affect the ratio of the precapillary resistance and the postcapillary resistance, and change the blood pressure in the capillary and the distribution of the body fluid within the vascular space.

10.1.7 Capacitance Vessel

Compared to the corresponding arteries, veins have a greater quantity, a thicker caliber, and a thinner vein wall. Therefore, the volume of the vein is larger and it has high expandability. Smaller pressure changes can make venous volume change considerably. At rest, the circulating blood volume of 60% to 70% is present in the vein. When the vein caliber changes slightly, the amount of blood that is injected into the vein can vary greatly. Veins play a role as a blood bank in the cardiovascular system and are called capacitance vessel.

10.1.8 Shunt Vessel

There are direct connections between arterioles and venules, called shunt vessels. Shunt vessels can make the blood in the arterioles flow directly into the venules without passing through the capillaries. There are many shunt vessels in the skin of the finger, the toe and the auricula, which are related to thermoregulation in function.

10.2 Resistance of Blood Flow

Resistance of blood flow originates from the frictional resistance between blood components (i.e., the viscosity of blood) and the frictional resistance between blood flow and the vascular wall. Due to resistance of blood flow, blood pressure will gradually decrease when blood flows through the blood vessels.

Resistance of blood flow is directly proportional to the length of the blood vessel and the viscosity of the blood, but is inversely proportional to the 4th power of the blood vessel radius. The resistance of blood flow is mainly determined by the radius of blood vessels and the viscosity of blood.

10.3 Blood Pressure

Blood pressure is the pressure of blood flow on the wall of a unit area. The measurement unit of blood pressure is **Pascal** (Pa, 帕), **kilopascal** (kPa, 千帕) and mmHg, and 1mmHg equals 0.133kPa. Venous blood pressure and atrial pressure are lower, and the measurement unit is cmH_2O, and $1cmH_2O$ equals 0.098kPa.

10.3.1 Measurement of Arterial Pressure

Recall that the systemic arterial pressure fluctuates with each heart cycle between a diastolic pressure and a higher systolic pressure. Obtaining estimates of systolic and diastolic pressures is one of the most routine diagnostic techniques available to the physician.

An inflatable cuff is wrapped around the upper arm, and a device, such as a mercury manometer, is attached to monitor the pressure within the cuff. The cuff is initially inflated with air to a pressure (175 to 200mmHg) that is well above normal systolic pressure. This pressure is transmitted from the flexible cuff into the upper arm, where it causes all blood vessels to collapse. No blood flows into (or out of) the forearm as long as the cuff pressure is higher than the systolic pressure. After the initial inflation, air is allowed to gradually "bleed" from the cuff so that the pressure within it falls slowly and steadily through the range of arterial pressure fluctuations. The moment the cuff pressure falls below the peak

systolic pressure, some blood is able to pass through the arteries beneath the cuff during the systolic phase of the cycle. This flow is intermittent and occurs only for a brief period during each heart cycle. Moreover, because it occurs through partially collapsed vessels beneath the cuff, the flow is turbulent rather than laminar. The intermittent periods of flow beneath the cuff produce tapping sounds, which can be detected with a stethoscope placed over the brachial artery at the elbow. Sounds of varying character, known collectively as Korotkoff sounds are heard whenever the cuff pressure is between the systolic and diastolic aortic pressures.

Because there is no blood flow and thus no sound when cuff pressure is higher than systolic pressure, the highest cuff pressure at which tapping sounds are heard is taken as the systolic pressure. When the cuff pressure falls below the diastolic pressure, blood flows through the vessels beneath the cuff without interruption and no sound is detected over the radial artery. The cuff pressure at which the sounds become muffled or disappear is taken as the diastolic pressure. The Korotkoff sounds are more distinct when the cuff pressure is near the systolic pressure than when it is near the diastolic pressure. Thus, consistency in determining diastolic pressure by auscultation requires concentration and experience.

10.3.2 Mean Arterial Pressure

Mean arterial pressure is a critically important cardiovascular variable because it is the average effective pressure that drives blood through the systemic organs. Most often, however, we know information about the systolic and diastolic pressures from auscultation only. Mean arterial pressure necessarily falls between the systolic and diastolic pressures. A useful rule of thumb is that mean arterial pressure is approximately equal to diastolic pressure plus one-third of the difference between systolic and diastolic pressure.

10.3.3 Arterial Pulse Pressure

The arterial pulse pressure is defined as systolic pressure minus diastolic pressure. Arterial pulse pressure is about 40mmHg in a normal resting young adult. Pulse pressure tends to increase with age in adults because of a decrease in arterial compliance (hardening of the arteries).

10.4 Formation of Arterial Blood Pressure

The basic condition for the formation of arterial blood pressure is that the circulatory system has sufficient blood volume, cardiac ejection, peripheral resistance and extensibility of windkessel vessels.

10.4.1 Enough Blood Filled Circulatory System

Sufficient blood volume in the circulatory system is the prerequisite for the formation of arterial blood pressure. The degree of blood filling in the circulatory system can be expressed by the mean circulatory filling pressure. The mean circulatory filling pressure is determined by the ratio between the circulating blood volume and the vascular system capacity. If the circulation blood volume increases or the vascular system capacity decreases, the mean circulatory filling pressure increases. Conversely, if the circulating blood volume decreases or the vascular system capacity increases, the mean circulatory filling pressure decreases.

10.4.2 Cardiac Ejection & Peripheral Resistance

Ventricular contraction and ejection make blood enter the vascular system overcoming peripheral resistance. The energy released by ventricular contraction can be divided into two parts, one is the kinetic energy that drives blood flow, and the other is the pressure on the blood vessel wall, that is, the pressure energy.

10.4.3 Extensibility of Windkessel Vessel

Cardiac ejection is interrupted, but blood flow in the circulatory system is continuous. Owing to the extensibility of the windkessel vessel, only 1/3 of the blood which ejected from the left ventricle flows into the peripheral vessels. The 2/3 of the blood which ejected from the left ventricle is temporarily stored in the windkessel vessel. So the speed and amplitude of aortic pressure increase are buffered. When the ventricle diastole, the dilated aorta retracts and continues to push the blood flow to the peripheral blood vessels, so that the aorta pressure can still be maintained at a high level. The expandability of the windkessel vessel is buffering the fluctuation of arterial blood pressure.

10.5 Influences on Arterial Blood Pressure

For convenience of discussion, in the following analysis, the effects of a factor on arterial blood pressure will be analyzed separately while keeping other conditions unchanged.

10.5.1 Stroke Volume

If stroke volume increases, the volume of blood ejected into the aorta during systole increases, and the increase of systolic pressure is more obvious. As the arterial blood pressure increases, the blood flow speeds up. Most of the increased blood volume in the aorta

can flow into the peripheral vessels in the diastolic phase. At the end of the diastole, the increase of blood stored in the aorta is lower than the increase in stroke volume. The arterial blood pressure is mainly manifested as the systolic pressure increases significantly, while the increasing level of diastolic pressure is relatively small, so the pulse pressure increases. Under normal circumstances, the level of systolic pressure mainly reflects the level of stroke volume.

10.5.2 Heart Rate

When the heart rate is accelerated, diastolic phase is significantly shortened, and blood flow into the peripheral vessels during diastolic phase is decreased. At the end of the diastolic phase, the blood volume in the aorta is increased and the diastolic pressure is increased. As the amount of blood stored in the aorta increases during systolic phase, the systolic pressure increases correspondingly. An increase in arterial blood pressure speeds up blood flow, and more blood flows into peripheral vessels during systolic phase. Therefore, the increase of systolic pressure is not as significant as that of diastolic pressure, and pulse pressure decreases.

10.5.3 Peripheral Resistance

When the peripheral resistance is accelerated, blood flow into the peripheral vessels during diastolic phase is decreased. At the end of the diastolic phase, the blood volume in the aorta increases and the diastolic pressure increases. As the amount of blood stored in the aorta increases during systolic phase, the systolic pressure increases correspondingly. An increase in arterial blood pressure speeds up blood flow, and more blood flows into peripheral vessels during systolic phase. Therefore, the increase in systolic pressure is not as significant as that of diastolic pressure, and pulse pressure decreases. Under normal circumstances, the level of diastolic pressure mainly reflects the level of peripheral resistance.

10.5.4 Extensibility of Windkessel Vessel

The expandability of the windkessel vessel is buffering the fluctuation of arterial blood pressure. Because of arteriosclerosis, the expandability of the windkessel vessel decreases, the systolic pressure rises, the diastolic pressure decreases, and the pulse pressure increases.

10.5.5 Mean Circulatory Filling Pressure

The mean circulatory filling pressure is determined by the ratio between the circulating blood volume and the vascular system capacity. If the circulation blood volume increases or the vascular system capacity decreases, the mean circulatory filling pressure increased. Conversely, if the circulating blood volume decreases or the vascular system capacity increases, the mean circulatory filling pressure decreases.

10.6 Venous Pressure

When the blood of systemic circulation reaches the vein, the blood pressure drops to 15–20mmHg. The right atrium is the endpoint of the systemic circulation, and the blood pressure is close to zero. The blood pressure in the right atrium and the large veins in the thoracic cavity is called **central venous pressure** (中心静脉压). The venous pressure of the organs is called peripheral venous pressure. The level of central venous pressure depends on the ability of cardiac ejection and venous blood volume. If the ventricular contractility is enhanced, the ventricular blood can be ejected into the artery in time, and the central venous pressure will be lower. On the contrary, if the ventricular contractility decreases, the central venous pressure rises. On the other hand, if the venous return increases, the central venous pressure will also increase. Therefore, central venous pressure is an important indicator of cardiovascular function. Central venous pressure is always inherently driven to the value that makes cardiac output and venous return equal.

Summary

体循环和肺循环的血管系统都由动脉、毛细血管和静脉所组成，动脉、毛细血管和静脉之间呈串联关系。从生理功能上可将血管分为以下几类：弹性储器血管、分配血管、毛细血管前阻力血管、毛细血管前括约肌、交换血管、毛细血管后阻力血管、容量血管和短路血管。

血液在血管内流动时所遇到的阻力，称为血流阻力。血流阻力使血液在血管内流动时压力逐渐降低。

血压是指流动着的血液对于单位面积血管壁的侧压力。在临床上，常用听诊法间接测定肱动脉的收缩压和舒张压。循环系统内的血液充盈、心脏射血和外周阻力，以及主动脉与大动脉的弹性储器作用是形成动脉血压的基本条件。

心室收缩时，主动脉压升高，在收缩期的中期达到最高值，此时的动脉血压值称为收缩压。心室舒张时，主动脉压下降，在心舒末期动脉血压的最低值称为舒张压。收缩压和舒张压的差值称为脉搏压，简称脉压。一个心动周期中每一瞬间动脉血压的平均值称为平均动脉压，平均动脉压约等于舒张压与1/3脉压之和。

影响动脉血压的因素：心脏搏出量、心率、外周阻力、主动脉和大动脉的弹性储器作用和循环血量与血管系统容量的比例。

通常将右心房和胸腔内大静脉的血压称为中心静脉压，而各器官静脉的血压则称为外周静脉压。中心静脉压的高低取决于心脏射血的能力和静脉回心血量之间的相互关系。

Xiao Yu (肖宇)

Chapter 11   Regulation of Arterial Pressure

Arterial pressure is continuously monitored by various sensors located within the body. Whenever arterial pressure varies from normal, multiple reflex responses are initiated which cause the adjustments in cardiac output and total peripheral resistance needed to return arterial pressure to its normal value. In the short-term regulation of arterial pressure, these adjustments are brought about by changes in the activity of the autonomic nerves leading to the heart and peripheral vessels. In the long-term regulation of arterial pressure, other mechanisms such as changes in cardiac output brought about by changes in blood volume play an increasingly important role in the control of arterial pressure.

11.1   Arterial Baroreceptor Reflex

The arterial baroreceptor reflex is the most important mechanism providing short-term regulation of arterial pressure. The usual components of the reflex arc include sensory receptors, afferent nerves, integrating centers in the central nervous system, efferent nerves, and effector organs. The efferent pathways of the arterial baroreceptor reflex are the cardiac sympathetic nerves, sympathetic vasoconstrictor nerves and cardiac parasympathetic nerves. The effector organs involved in this reflex are the heart and peripheral blood vessels.

11.1.1   Efferent Pathways

1) Cardiac Sympathetic Nerve and Function: The preganglionic neurons of the cardiac sympathetic nerve are located in the thoracic 1–5 segment of the spinal cord. The postganglionic fibers of cardiac sympathetic nerve innervate various parts of the heart, including sinoatrial node, atrioventricular junction atrioventricular bundle, atrial myocardium and ven-

tricular muscle. The sympathetic fibers innervating the sinoatrial node mainly come from the right cardiac sympathetic nerve, so the excitation of the right cardiac sympathetic nerve mainly causes the heart rate to increase. The sympathetic fibers innervating the atrioventricular junction and ventricular muscle mainly come from the left cardiac sympathetic nerve, so the excitation of the left cardiac sympathetic nerve mainly causes myocardial contractility to increase.

Norepinephrine released from postganglionic fibers of cardiac sympathetic nerve can accelerate heart rate, accelerate atrioventricular conduction, and enhance the contractility of atrial and ventricular muscles, resulting in the positive chronotropic action, the positive dromotropic action and the positive inotropic action. These actions are mainly due to the activation of the β_1 adrenergic receptor on the myocardial cell membrane by norepinephrine.

2) Cardiac Vagus Nerve and Function: The preganglionic neurons of the cardiac vagus nerve are located in the dorsal nucleus and nucleus of the vagus nerve in the medulla oblongata. The postganglionic fibers of cardiac vagus nerve innervate various parts of the heart, including the sinoatrial node, atrioventricular junction, atrioventricular bundle, and atrial myocardium. The parasympathetic fibers innervating the sinoatrial node mainly come from the right cardiac vagus nerve. The parasympathetic fibers innervating the atrioventricular junction mainly come from the left cardiac vagus nerve.

Acetylcholine released from postganglionic fibers of cardiac vagus nerve can cause the heart rate slowing down, the atrioventricular conduction slows, and the atrial muscle contraction abate, that is, the negative chronotropic action, the negative dromotropic action and the negative inotropic action. These actions are mainly due to the activation of the M type cholinergic receptor on the myocardial cell membrane by acetylcholine.

3) Sympathetic Vasoconstrictor Nerve Fibers and Function: The preganglionic neurons of the sympathetic vasoconstrictor nerve fibers are located in the thoracic spinal cord and lumbar spinal cord. The postganglionic fibers of the sympathetic vasoconstrictor nerve fibers innervate vascular smooth muscle cell.

Acetylcholine is released from preganglionic fibers of sympathetic vasoconstrictor nerve fibers. Norepinephrine is released from postganglionic fibers of sympathetic vasoconstrictor nerve fibers. When norepinephrine is combined with α receptor, the vascular smooth muscle can be contracted. When combined with the β_2 receptor, the vascular smooth muscle relaxes. However, the ability of norepinephrine to combine with β_2 receptor is weak. Therefore, vasoconstriction is the main action of the sympathetic vasoconstrictor nerve fibers.

11.1.2　Sensory Receptors

Sensory receptors, called arterial baroreceptors are found in abundance in the walls of the aorta and carotid arteries. Sensory receptors are found near the arch of the aorta which called the aortic baroreceptors. Sensory receptors are found near the point where carotid artery divides into the internal carotid artery and the external carotid artery, which are called the carotid sinus baroreceptors.

The receptors themselves are mechanoreceptors that sense arterial pressure indirectly by detecting the degree of stretch in the elastic arterial walls. In general, increased stretch causes an increased actionpotentials generation rate by the arterial baroreceptors. Baroreceptors actually sense not only absolute stretch but also the rate of change in stretch. For this reason, both the mean arterial pressure and arterial pulse pressure affect baroreceptor firing rate. Note that the presence of pulsations increases the baroreceptor firing rate at any given level of mean arterial pressure. Note also that small changes in mean arterial pressure near the normal value of 100mmHg produce the largest changes in baroreceptor discharge rate.

If arterial pressure remains elevated over a period of several days for some reason, the arterial baroreceptor firing rate will gradually return toward normal. Thus, arterial baroreceptors are said to adapt to long-term changes in arterial pressure. For this reason, the arterial baroreceptor reflex cannot serve as a mechanism for the long-term regulation of arterial pressure.

11.1.3　Afferent Pathways

Action potentials generated by the carotid sinus baroreceptors travel through the carotid sinus nerves, which join with the glossopharyngeal nerves before entering the central nervous system. Afferent fibers from the aortic baroreceptors run to the central nervous system in the vagus nerves. The vagus nerves contain both afferent and efferent fibers.

11.1.4　Central Integration

Much of the central integration involved in reflex regulation of the cardiovascular system occurs in the medulla oblongata where are traditionally referred to as the medullary cardiovascular centers. The neural interconnections between the diffuse structures in this area are complex and not completely mapped. Moreover, these structures appear to serve multiple functions including respiratory control. For example, what is known with a fair degree of certainty is where the cardiovascular afferent and efferent pathways enter and leave the medulla. The afferent sensory information from the arterial baroreceptors enters the nucleus tractus solitarius in the medulla, where it is relayed via polysynaptic pathways to other structures. The cell bodies of the efferent vagal parasympathetic cardiac nerves are located primarily in the medullary nucleus ambiguus. The sympathetic autonomic efferent information leaves the medulla predominantly from the rostral ventrolateral medulla group of neurons via an excitatory spinal pathway or via the raphe nucleus through an inhibitory spinal pathway.

11.1.5　Operation of Arterial Baroreceptor Reflex

The arterial baroreceptor reflex Fig. 11-1 is a continuously operating control system that automatically makes adjustments to prevent disturbances on the heart and/or vessels from causing large changes in mean arterial pressure. The arterial baroreceptor reflex mechanism acts to regulate arterial pressure in a negative feedback manner that is analogous in many ways to the manner in which a thermostatically controlled home heating system operates to regulate inside temperature despite disturbances such as changes in the weather or open windows.

Fig. 11-1 shows many events in the arterial baroreceptor reflex pathway that occur in response to a disturbance of decreased mean arterial pressure. All of the events shown in Fig. 11-1 have already been discussed, and each should be carefully examined (and reviewed if necessary) at this point because a great many of the interactions that are essential to understanding cardiovascular physiology are summarized in this figure.

11.2　Reflexes from Receptors in Heart & Lungs

A host of mechanoreceptors and chemoreceptors that can elicit reflex cardiovascular responses have been identified in the atria, ventricles, coronary vessels, and lungs. The role of these cardiopulmonary receptors in the neurohumoral control of the cardiovascular system is, in most cases, incompletely understood, but evidence is accumulating that they may be involved significantly in many physiological and pathological states.

One general function that the cardiopulmonary receptors perform is sensing the pressure (or volume) in the atria and central venous pool. Increased central venous pressure and volume causes receptor activation by stretch, which elicits a reflex decrease in sympathetic activity. Decreased central venous pressure produces the opposite response. Volume receptor reflex normally exert a tonic inhibitory influence on sympathetic activity and play an arguably important role in normal cardiovascular regulation.

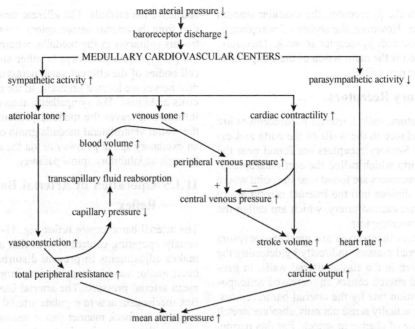

Figure 11-1   Immediate cardiovascular adjustments caused by a decrease in arterial blood pressure.

11.3   Chemoreceptor Reflex

Low PO_2 and/or high PCO_2 levels in the arterial blood cause reflex increments in respiratory rate and mean arterial pressure. This appears to be a result of increased activity of peripheral chemoreceptors, located in the carotid arteries and the arch of the aorta, and central chemoreceptors, located somewhere within the central nervous system. Peripheral chemoreceptors probably play little role in the normal regulation of arterial pressure because arterial blood PO_2 and PCO_2 are normally held very nearly constant by respiratory control mechanisms.

11.4   Fluid Balance & Arterial Pressure

Several key factors in the long-term regulation of arterial blood pressure have already been considered. The first fact is the fact that the baroreceptor reflex, however well, it counteracts temporary disturbances in arterial pressure, cannot effectively regulate arterial pressure in the long term for the simple reason that the baroreceptor firing rate adapts to prolonged changes in arterial pressure.

The second pertinent fact is that circulating blood volume can influence arterial pressure because:

Blood volume↓
↓
Peripheral venous pressure↓
↓
Left shift of venous function curve↓
↓

Central venous pressure↓
↓
Cardiac output↓
↓
Arterial pressure↓

A fact yet to be considered is that arterial pressure has a profound influence on urinary output rate and thus affects total body fluid volume. Because blood volume is one of the components of the total body fluid, blood volume alterations accompany changes in total body fluid volume. The mechanisms are such that an increase in arterial pressure causes an increase in urinary output rate and thus a decrease in blood volume. But, as outlined in the preceding sequence, decreased blood volume tends to lower arterial pressure. Thus, the complete sequence of events that are initiated by an increase in arterial pressure can be listed as follows:

Arterial pressure (disturbance)↑
↓
Urinary output rate↑
↓
Fluid volume↓
↓
Blood volume↓
↓
Cardiac output↓
↓
Arterial pressure (compensation)↓

Note the negative feedback nature of this sequence of events: increased arterial pressure leads to fluid volume depletion, which tends to lower arterial pressure. Conversely, an initial disturbance of decreased arterial pressure would lead to fluid volume expansion, which would tend to increase arterial pressure. Because of negative feedback, these events constitute a fluid volume mechanism for regulating arterial pressure.

Summary

　　人体在不同的生理状况下，各器官组织的代谢水平不同，对血流量的需要也不同。机体可通过神经和体液机制对心脏和各部分血管的活动进行调节，从而适应各器官组织在不同情况下对血流量的需要，协调地进行各器官之间的血流分配。心肌和血管平滑肌都接受自主神经的支配，机体对心血管活动的神经调节是通过各种心血管反射实现的。

　　心交感神经节后纤维末梢释放的去甲肾上腺素可引起心率加快，房室传导加快，心房肌和心室肌收缩力加强，即产生正性变时作用、正性变传导作用和正性变力作用。这些作用主要是由于去甲肾上腺素激活了心肌细胞膜上的β_1肾上腺素能受体引起的。

　　心迷走神经节后纤维末梢释放的乙酰胆碱作用于心肌细胞膜上的M型胆碱能受体（M受体）后可引起心率减慢，房室传导减慢，心房肌收缩能力减弱，即产生负性变时作用、负性变传导作用和负性变力作用。心迷走神经的负性变力作用主要表现在心房肌，对心室肌作用不大。

　　交感缩血管神经纤维末梢释放去甲肾上腺素。去甲肾上腺素与α受体结合后，可使血管平滑肌收缩；而与β_2受体结合后，则使血管平滑肌舒张。但是，去甲肾上腺素与β_2受体结合的能力较弱。因此，缩血管纤维兴奋时主要引起缩血管效应。

　　动脉血压升高时，压力感受器传入冲动增多，通过有关的心血管中枢整合作用，使心迷走紧张加强，心交感紧张和交感缩血管紧张降低，其效应为心率减慢，心输出量减少，外周血管阻力降低，故动脉血压回降。反之，当动脉血压降低时，压力感受器传入冲动减少，使迷走紧张降低，交感紧张加强，于是心率加快，心输出量增加，外周血管阻力增高，血压回升。

　　根据各种神经、体液因素对动脉血压调节的时程，可将动脉血压调节分为短期调节和长期调节。短期调节是指对短时间内发生的血压变化起即刻调节作用，主要是神经调节，包括各种心血管反射通过调节心肌收缩力和血管外周阻力使动脉血压恢复正常并保持相对稳定，其具体机制如前述。而当血压在较长时间内（数小时、数天、数月或更长）发生变化时，单纯依靠神经调节常不足以将血压调节到正常水平。动脉血压的长期调节主要是通过肾脏调节细胞外液量来实现的，因而构成肾-体液控制系统。当体内细胞外液量增多时，循环血量增多，循环血量和血管系统容量之间的相对关系发生改变，使动脉血压升高；而循环血量增多和动脉血压升高，又能直接导致肾排水和排钠增加，将过多的体液排出体外，从而使血压恢复到正常水平。当体内细胞外液量或循环血量减少，血压下降时，则发生相反的调节。

Xiao Yu (肖宇)

Part Ⅳ   Pathologic Circulatory System

Chapter 12   Pathologic Circulatory System

OUTLINE

12.1 General Description

12.2 Atherosclerosis

12.3 Hypertension

12.4 Rheumatism

12.5 Infective Endocarditis

12.1 General Description

The circulatory system is an organ system that permits blood and lymph circulation to transport nutrients (such as amino acids and electrolytes), oxygen, carbon dioxide, hormones, blood cells, etc. It nourishes cells in the body, helps to fight diseases, stabilizes body temperature and pH, and maintains homeostasis.

Cardiovascular diseases comprise the most prevalent serious disorders in industrialized countries and are a rapidly growing problem in developing countries. Age-adjusted mortality for coronary heart disease has declined by two-thirds in the past four decades in the United States, reflecting the identification and reduction of risk factors as well as improved treatments and interventions for heart failure. Nonetheless, cardiovascular diseases remain the most common cause of death, responsible for 35% of all deaths, almost 1 million deaths each year. Approximately one-fourth of these deaths are sudden.

In addition, cardiovascular diseases are highly prevalent. 80 million adults are diagnosed and it takes up 35% of the adult population. For many years cardiovascular disease was considered to be more common in men than in women. In fact, women die from cardiovascular diseases at a higher rate than men.

Coronary artery disease (CAD) is more frequently associated with dysfunction of the coronary microcirculation in women than in men. Exercise induced myocardial infarction is more common in women than in men.

12.2 Atherosclerosis

Arteriosclerosis (动脉粥样硬化) is a generic, inclusive term that describes thickening and hardening of the arterial wall. This term includes three pathologic entities: atherosclerosis, arteriosclerosis and arterial medial calcification.

Atherosclerosis is a multifactorial degenerative disease characterized by the formation of plaques on the intima. These lesions are called atheromas (or atheromatous or atherosclerotic plaques). Atheromatous plaques are raised lesions composed of soft gummous lipid cores (mainly cholesterol and cholesterol esters, with necrotic debris) covered by fibrous caps.

Arteriolosclerosis affects small arteries and arterioles. The two anatomic variants, hyalinosis and hyperplasia, are both associated with vessel wall thickening and luminal narrowing that may cause downstream ischemic injury.

This disease is commonly found in every adult over the age of 40, as well as in many younger individuals. Large and medium-sized arteries are usually involved.

12.2.1 Etiology and Pathogenesis

12.2.1.1 Etiology

The prevalence and severity of atherosclerosis and **ischemic heart disease** (IHD, 缺血性心脏病) among individuals and groups are related to several risk factors, some constitutional, but others acquired or related to behaviors and potentially amenable to manipulation. Risk factors have been identified through a number of prospective studies in well-defined populations, particularly the Framingham Heart Study and Atherosclerosis Risk in Communities. The risk factors are as follows:

1) Hyperlipidemia (高脂血症): It is a major risk factor for the development of atherosclerosis. The main cholesterol component associated with increased risk is low-density lipoprotein (LDL) cholesterol. By contrast, high-density lipoprotein (HDL) mobilizes cholesterol from developing and existing vascular plaques and transporting it to the liver for biliary excretion. Consequently, higher levels of HDL correlate with lower risk.

2) Hypertension (高血压): Hypertension is another major risk factor for development of atherosclerosis. Hypertension can increase the risk of IHD by approximately 60%. Hypertension is also the major cause of left ventricular hypertrophy (LVH), which also can contribute to myocardial ischemia. There is a close relationship between hypertension and atherosclerosis, with mutual influence and mutual promotion. Hypertension is similar to atherosclerosis pathologic changes, such as inflammatory responses of blood vessel wall, damage of endothelial cells, etc.

3) Smoking: It is a well-established risk factor. Prolonged smoking of one or more packs of cigarettes a day doubles the rate of IHD-related mortality. Smoking, whether active, exposed, or passive, increases the risk of cardiovascular disease.

The smoke composition is complex, contains many kinds of harmful substances to the human body, high concentration of carbon monoxide can induce arrhythmia. Nicotine can cause vasoconstriction, thin tube cavity and increased vascular resistance, leading to hypertension. The most effective method is to quit smoking, and the risk of coronary heart disease can be reduced by 50% after a year.

4) Diabetes mellitus (糖尿病): Diabetes mellitus is associated with hypercholesterolemia as well as a markedly increased predisposition to atherosclerosis. Other factors being equal, the incidence of arteriosclerosis is twice as high in diabetic patients as compared to non-diabetic individuals. There is also a 100-fold increased risk of atherosclerosis-induced gangrene of the lower extremities.

5) Genetics (遗传): Family history is the most important independent risk factor for atherosclerosis. Most familial risks are related to polygenic traits that go hand-in-hand with atherosclerosis, such as hypertension and diabetes, as well as other genetic polymorphisms.

The well-established familial predisposition to atherosclerosis and IHD is multifactorial. In some instances, it relates to familial clustering of other risk factors, such as hypertension or diabetes, whereas in others, it involves well-defined genetic derangements in lipoprotein metabolism, such as familial hypercholesterolemia, that result in excessively high blood lipid levels.

6) Age and gender: Age is a dominant influence. Although the accumulation of atherosclerotic plaque is typically a progressive process, it does not usually manifest clinically until lesions reach a critical threshold and begin to precipitate organ injury in middle age or later. Thus, between ages 40 and 60, the incidence of myocardial infarction in men increases fivefold, even though the underlying arterial lesions are probably evolving before that. Death rates from IHD rise with each decade, even into advanced age.

Premenopausal women have a lower incidence than men of the same age. Women have higher HDL levels and lower LDL levels than men because estrogen has the function of altering the endothelium of the blood vessel and lowering blood cholesterol levels. This difference disappears after menopause.

12.2.1.2   Pathogenesis

The overwhelming clinical importance of atherosclerosis has stimulated enormous efforts to understand its cause. The contemporary view of atherogenesis is expressed by the response-to-injury hypothesis. This model views atherosclerosis as a chronic inflammatory response of the arterial wall to endothelial injury. Lesion progression occurs through interactions of modified lipoproteins, monocyte-derived macrophages, T lymphocytes, and the normal cellular constituents of the arterial wall. The followings are central tenets of the hypothesis.

1) Lipid infiltration: Chronic endothelial injury, with resultant endothelial dysfunction, causes increased permeability, leukocyte adhesion, and thrombosis. Lipoproteins accumulate in the vessel wall and monocytes adhere to the endothelium, followed by migration into the intima and transformation into macrophages and foam cells. Platelet adhesion factors released from activated platelets, macrophages, and vascular wall cells induce smooth muscle cell (SMC) recruitment, SMC proliferation and extracellular matrix (ECM) production either from the media or from circulating precursors. Lipids accumulate both extracellularly and within cells. Lipids are typically transported in the blood stream binding to mutations in genes. Dyslipidemia can result from mutations in genes that encode apolipoproteins, lipoprotein receptors, or from disorders that derange lipid metabolism.

The mechanisms by which dyslipidemia contributes to atherogenesis include the following: chronic hyperlipidemia, particularly hypercholesterolemia, can directly impair endothelial cell function by increasing local oxygen free radical production. In addition, oxygen free radicals accelerate nitric oxide (NO) decay, damping its vasodilator activity.

With chronic hyperlipidemia, lipoproteins accumulate within the intima, where they are hypothesized to generate two pathogenic derivatives, oxidized LDL and cholesterol crystals.

2) Response to injury hypothesis: Chronic or repetitive endothelial injury is the cornerstone of the response-to-injury hypothesis. Endothelial loss due to any kind of injury, whether induced experimentally by mechanical denudation, hemodynamic forces, immune complex deposition, irradiation, or chemicals-results in intimal thickening; in the presence of high-lipid diets, typical atheromas ensue. After vascular endothelial cell injury, atherosclerosis is mainly caused by the following links.

① **Vascular wall barrier dysfunction:** After vascular endothelial cell injury, endothelial cell death leads to the destruction of intimal integrity or endothelial function. Obstruction leads to an increased intercellular space and barrier function.

There is a lipid concentration between the blood and the walls of the blood vessel. Vascular endothelial cells enhance the capacity of the lipid in the blood, which together promote the lipids in the blood to enter the vessel wall deposition, resulting in atherosclerosis.

② **Anti-adhesion dysfunction:** When endothelial cells are damaged, the surface adhesion molecules are increased, or the subcutaneous material are directly in contact with the blood, resulting in an increase of platelets, monocytes, neutrophils and other adhesions in the blood, which in turn leads to thrombosis and inflammatory response.

③ **Endocrine system impairment:** The vascular system, including vascular endothelial cells and smooth muscle cells, is considered to be one of the largest endocrine tissues in the human body. It has endocrine function.

Vasoactive substances play a vital role in maintaining normal function and homeostasis of blood vessels.

Risk factors of atherosclerosis often cause endothelial cell dysfunction, vasoconstriction and diastolic dysfunction, promote or inhibit SMC growth, and so on, thereby promoting the development of atherosclerosis.

3) Smooth Muscle Proliferation: Intimal SMC proliferation and ECM deposition convert a fatty streak into a mature atheroma and contribute to the progressive growth of atherosclerotic lesions. Several growth factors are implicated in SMC proliferation and ECM synthesis, including platelet-derived growth factor, fibroblast growth factor, and transforming growth factor α.

Several growth factors are implicated in SMC proliferation and ECM synthesis, including platelet-derived growth factor. The recruited SMCs synthesize ECM (most notably collagen), which stabilizes atherosclerotic SMC apoptosis and breakdown of matrix, leading to the development of unstable plaques.

4) Inflammation (炎症): Inflammatory cells and mediators are involved in the initiation, progression, and the complications of atherosclerotic lesions. Although normal vessels do not bind to inflammatory cells, ECS in early atherogenesis express adhesion molecules that encourage leukocyte adhesion; vascular cell adhesion molecule 1 (VCAM-1) in particular binds to monocytes and T cells. After these cells adhere to the endothelium, they migrate into the intima under the influence of locally produced chemokines.

Monocytes differentiate into macrophages and avidly engulf lipoproteins, including oxidized LDL and small cholesterol crystals. Cholesterol crystals appear to be particularly important instigators of inflammation through activation of the inflammasome and

subsequent release of IL-1. T lymphocytes recruited to the intima interact with the macrophages and also contribute to a state of chronic inflammation.

12.2.2 Morphology

12.2.2.1 Basic change

1) Fatty streaks (脂纹): Fatty streaks are composed of lipid-filled foam cells but are not significantly raised and thus do not cause any disturbance in blood flow. Fatty streaks begin as minute yellow, flat macules that coalesce into elongated lesions. The relationship of fatty streaks to atherosclerotic plaques is uncertain; although they may evolve into precursors of plaques, not all fatty streaks are destined to become advanced atherosclerotic lesions (Fig. 12-1). In electron microscopy, there are two kinds of foamy cells: one is macrophage-derived foam cell, and the other is smooth muscle-derived foam cell.

Foam cells are round and large in volume, with a large amount of lipid vacuoles in the cytoplasm. Most of them are macrophages.

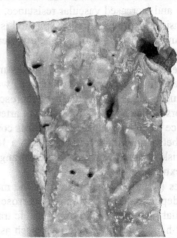

Figure 12-1 Severe atherosclerosis of the lower abdominal aorta. Note multiple areas of ulceration with adherent mural thrombus.

2) Fibrous plaque (纤维斑块): Fibrous plaques are developed from lipids. The term "fibrous plaque" refers to the gross morphologic appearance of the lesion that is the hallmark of the Acherosclerosis. Atheromatous plaques impinge on the lumen of the artery and grossly appear white to yellow; thrombosis superimposed over the surface of ulcerated plaques is red-brown in color.

In gross, the lesions are raised, pearly white to gray, smooth-surfaced, plaque-like structures in the intima that vary in diameter from a few millimeters to over a centimeter. Microscopically the surface of plaque is hyperplastic collagen fibers. The fibrous cap is composed of avascular connective tissues and elongated SMCs (Fig. 12-2). The central plaque consists of some foam cells and SMCs.

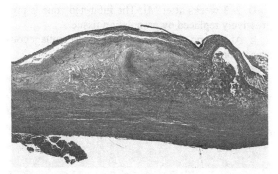

Figure 12-2   Atherosclerotic plaque.

3) Atheromatous plaque (atheroma) (粥样斑块):

It is a typical lesion of atherosclerosis. Atheromatous plaques are white to yellow raised lesions. Atherosclerotic plaques are patchy, usually involving only a portion of any given arterial wall. On cross section, therefore, the lesions appear "eccentric" (Fig. 12-3).

LM (light microscope):

① Surface: Fibrous cap hyaline degeneration of collagen;

② Necrotic center: Amorphous necrotic materials;

③ Surrounding: Granulation tissue, lipid cores (LC), and foam cells.

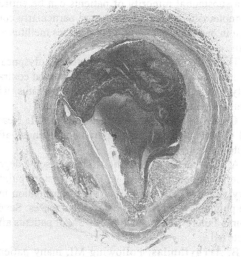

Figure 12-3   Coronary artery narrowing caused by atherosclerosis. Low magnification.

Plaques generally continue to change and progressively enlarge through cell death and degeneration, synthesis and degradation of ECM (remodeling), and thrombus organization. Atheromas also often undergo calcification.

12.2.2.2   Secondary lesions

Secondary lesions are common on the basis of fibrous plaques and atheromatous plaques.

1) Intraplaque hemorrhage: Rupture of new blood vessels in plaques creates haematoma, to further reduce and even completely occludethe lumen, causing acute blood loss.

2) Plaque rupture: A fibrous cap on the surface of the plaque breaks the atheroma and spreads from the fissure to the bloodstream, retained tumor like ulcer. Necrotic substances and lipids released into the bloodstream can form cholesterol emboli.

3) Thrombosis: Plaque ruptures and forms ulceration, due to collagen exposure, promotes blood clot formation, which causes obstruction of the artery cavity, leading to the infarction of the tube.

4) Calcification: In the fibrous cap and congee tumor lesions, the wall of calcium salt deposit is hardened and brittle.

5) Aneurysm formation: Atheromatous plaques can occur when the bottom of the smooth muscle has different degrees of atrophy and decreased elasticity. Under the action of internal pressure, the artery wall expands locally, forming aneurysm.

6) Vascular lumen: Muscular arteries can be caused by atherosclerotic plaques, resulting in lumen narrowing, reducing the area of blood supply, and resulting in ischemic lesions in the corresponding organs.

12.2.2.3   Atherosclerosis of aorta

Aortic atherosclerosis lesion occurs in the posterior wall of the aorta and its branching points, the abdominal aortic lesions are the most severe. However, due to the large active intracavicular, there is no obvious symptom caused by severe atherosclerosis. In severe cases, due to the contraction of the middle membrane and the rupture of the elastic plate, the lumen becomes weak and the blood pressure can easily form an aneurysm. The rupture of an aneurysm can be fatal.

12.2.2.4   Coronary atherosclerosis and coronary atherosclerotic heart disease

Coronary atherosclerosis is the most common disease in coronary arteries and is a serious disease that threatens human health. Coronary artery stenosis develops rapidly between the ages of 35 and 45. According to the detection rate and statistical results of the lesion, the anterior descending branch of the left coronary artery is of the highest incidence. The incidence decreases sequentially in the right trunk, left trunk or left-lateral branch, and the lower branch.

Coronary heart disease is caused by myocardial ischemia which is contributed by coronary artery stenosis, also known as ischemic heart disease. The most common cause is atherosclerosis in coronary arteries, which are closer to the ventricles of the heart than the other arteries. The coronary atherosclerosis is more severe than in other arteries. Main clinical manifestations include:

1) Angina pectoris (心绞痛): Angina pectoris is intermittent chest pain caused by transient, reversible myocardial ischemia. There are three types:

Typical angina: Typical angina also called stable angina, is an episodic chest pain associated with exertion or some other form of increased myocardial oxygen demand. The pain is classically described as a crushing or squeezing substernal sensation, which can radiate down the left arm or to the left shoulder.

Variant angina pectoris (known as prinzmetal angina): It usually occurs at rest due to coronary artery spasm. The etiology is not clear, but Prinzmetal angina typically responds promptly to the administration of vasodilators such as nitroglycerin or calcium channel blockers.

Unstable angina: It is more intense and longer lasting than stable angina. It is due to atherosclerotic plaque rupture or erosive thrombosis. Acute or subacute myocardial infarction is caused by vasoconstriction and microvascular embolism. Diffuse interstitial myocardial fibrosis is common.

2) Myocardial infarction (MI) (心肌梗死): It is necrosis of heart muscle resulting from ischemia. Roughly more than 1 million people in China die from MI every year. MI is extremely common, accounting for 10% to 15% of all deaths (Fig. 12-4).

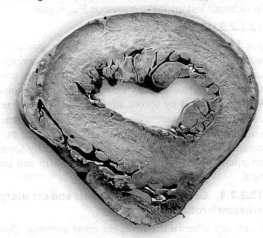

Figure 12-4 Myocardial infarction.

Nearly all transmural infarcts affect at least a portion of the left ventricle and ventricular septum. Significant atherosclerosis or thrombosis of penetrating intramyocardial branches of coronary arteries rarely occurs. MI can be divided into two types: regional myocardial infarction and transmural myocardial infarction (Fig. 12-5).
① **The pathological changes:** The morphological change of myocardial infarction is a dynamic process.

A. Within 4 to 12 hours: Typical characteristics of coagulative necrosis become detectable. "Wavy fibers" at the edges of an infarct reflect the stretching and buckling of noncontractile dead fibers but are considered "soft" findings of acute infarction.

B. 1–3 days after MI: Necrotic myocardium elicits acute inflammation.

C. 5–10 days after MI: A wave of macrophages to remove necrotic myocytes and neutrophil fragments.

D. 2–3 weeks after MI: The infarcted zone is progressively replaced by granulation tissue.

E. At the end of the sixth week dense collagenous scar is formed.

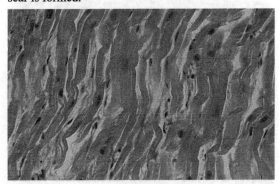

Figure 12-5 Acute myocardial infarction 1–3 days after onset.

② **Clinical features:** MI is usually heralded by severe, crushing substernal chest pain or discomfort that can radiate to the neck, jaw, epigastrium, or left arm. In contrast to the pain of angina pectoris, the pain of an MI typically lasts from 20min to several hours and is not significantly relieved by nitroglycerin or rest. In a substantial minority of patients can be entirely asymptomatic. These situations are particularly common in patients with underlying diabetes mellitus and in the elderly.

The pulse is generally rapid and weak, dyspnea is common and caused by impaired myocardial contractility, dysfunction of the mitral valve apparatus, with resultant pulmonary congestion and edema.
③ **Consequences and complications of MI:** Nearly 3/4 of patients have one or more complications after acute MI.

A. **Contractile dysfunction**: There is some degree of left ventricular failure, with hypotension, pulmonary vascular congestion, and fluid transudation into the pulmonary interstitial and alveolar spaces. Severe "pump failure" occurs in 10% to 15% of patients after acute MI.

B. **Arrhythmias**: Following MI, many patients develop arrhythmias, which undoubtedly are responsible for many of the sudden deaths.

C. **Pericarditis**: A fibrinous or hemorrhagic pericarditis usually develops within 2 to 3 days of a transmural MI.

D. **Mural thrombus**: For any infarct, the combination of a local loss of contractility with endocardial damage can foster mural thrombosis and thromboembolism potentially.

E. **Ventricular aneurysm**: Aneurysms of the ventricular wall most commonly result from a large transmural anteroseptal infarct that heals with the formation of thin scar tissue.

12.3   Hypertension

Hypertension is one of the most common serious cardiovascular diseases. Arterial hypertension is defined as a sustained rise of the systemic blood pressure above 140mmHg (18.4kPa) systolic and / or 90mmHg (12.0kPa) diastolic. Hypertension can be classified into two main types according to its etiology. Primary hypertension refers to elevation of blood pressure with age but with no apparent cause, secondary hypertension elevated blood pressure due to an identifiable cause. Hypertension disease means primary hypertension.

Primary hypertension is one of the most common cardiovascular diseases in China. In the vast majority of patients with hypertension, the underlying cause is unknown. Primary hypertension tends to be familial. The incidence of hypertension and its complication are different between gender and race. Males tend to have higher blood pressure than females of the same age before 55 years old. But at the age of 75, females tend to have higher hypertension incidence.

Secondary hypertension accounts for 5%–10% of hypertension. Special types of hypertension include pregnancy-associated hypertension and hypertension crisis by hypertensive encephalopathy, intracranial hemorrhage, unstable angina pectoris, acute myocardial infarction (AMI).

12.3.1   Etiology and Pathogenesis

So far the causes of hypertension are not clear. It is believed that hypertension is the result of interaction of genetic and environmental factors.

12.3.1.1   Risk factors

1) Genetic and familial aggregation: Genetic factors clearly play a role in determining pressure levels, as evidenced by studies. However, it is unlikely that a mutation at a single gene locus will engage as a major cause of essential hypertension.

High salt intake is thought to be an exogenous factor in hypertension. Obesity and drinking are one of the pathogenic factors of hypertension.

2) Environmental factors: Physical inactivity has been considered as exogenous factors in hypertension. Environmental factors affect the variables that control blood pressure in the genetically predisposed individuals.

12.3.1.2   Pathogenesis

1) The Na^+ and water retention caused by various mechanisms including genetic defect and genetic abnormality.
2) Abnormal peripheral vascular function, structure and contraction.
3) Peripheral vascular structure changes, peripheral resistance increases and blood pressure rises.

12.3.2   Morphology

According to pathological features, primary hypertension can be divided into two types, benign and malignant hypertension.

12.3.2.1   Benign hypertension

Benign hypertension is encountered in about 95% of hypertensive subjects. The patients are usually asymptomatic and the diagnosis is often made incidentally. With regard to the development of diseases, these patients fall into three phases.

1) Dysfunction: It is the early changes of hypertension. Arterioles show interval spasms. Blood pressure is increased accompanied by headache. However, blood pressure can return to normal after easing spasm.

2) Artery lesion: It is the characteristic lesion of hypertension. Under microscopy, the intimal SMCs proliferate. Such intimal proliferation is most often observed in renal arteries, one of the earliest changes noted in the wall of arteries. These lesions can be called hyaline arteriolosclerosis.

3) Viscera lesion

① **Heart:** The essential feature of hypertensive heart disease is left ventricular hypertrophy. The weight of the heart usually exceeds 400g. The hypertrophy typically involves the ventricular wall in a symmetric, circumferential pattern termed concentric hypertrophy. Musculi papillares and adductor are thickened. Microscopically, myocardial cells become thick and long, accompanied by more branching (Fig. 12-6). Nucleus of myocardial cell is large, round and dark.

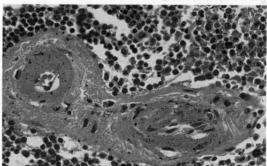

Figure 12-6   Vascular changes in malignant hypertension.

② **Kidney:** The hyaline and fibrous changes in blood vessels cause vascular narrowing and consequently lead to glomeruli ischemic atrophy and fibrosis, as well as tubular atrophy and interstitial fibrosis. Glomeruli compensatory hypertrophy and renal tubular compensatory enlargement can also occur. The kidneys may be normal in size or moderately reduced. The cortical surface is fine-grained, also called primary granular atrophy of the kidney. The cut section shows cortical thinning and the boundary of renal cortex and medulla is unclear.

③ **Brain**: In high blood pressure, a series of brain changes can occur as a result of small arterial spasms and sclerosis in the brain. **Hypertensive encephalopathy** (高血压脑病): The clinical features of acute hypertensive encephalopathy include headache, nausea, vomiting and reduced consciousness. Two reasons can explain the pathogenesis of acute hypertensive encephalopathy. Firstly, it is due to cerebral vasospasm with subsequent focal cerebral ischemia. Secondly, it is caused by over stretching of the arteriolar walls with extravasation of plasma proteins. **Cerebromalacia** (脑软化): Atherosclerosis in small arteries leads to cerebral ischemia, forming microinfarcts. It can affect small areas. After a few weeks or months, the necrotic tissue fades away and is repaired with a glial scar. **Cerebral hemorrhage** (脑出血): It is a serious and life-threatening complication. Hypertension is the most common underlying cause of intraparenchymal hemorrhages, and brain hemorrhage accounts for roughly 15% of deaths among individuals with chronic hypertension. Hypertensive intraparenchymal hemorrhages typically occur in the basal ganglia thalamus, pons, and cerebellum.

12.3.2.2 Malignant hypertension

It tends to occur in young adults. Blood pressure rises significantly, often over 230/130mmHg. The pathognomonic lesions of malignant hypertension are proliferative endarteritis and hyperplastic arteriolosclerosis. Vessels exhibit "onion skin" concentric, laminated thickening of arteriolar walls and luminal narrowing. In malignant hypertension, these changes are accompanied by fibrinoid deposits and vessel wall necrosis which is particularly prominent in the kidney.

12.4　Rheumatism

Rheumatism (风湿病) is a disease of disordered immunity characterized by inflammatory changes in the heart and joints, and in some cases associated with neurological symptoms. It is an acute, recurrent, inflammatory disease occuring most often in adolescents. Etiology and pathogenesis remain unclear.

Acute rheumatic fever (RF) is closely related to infection with streptococci group A. It is a hypersensitivity reaction induced by host antibodies elicited by streptococci group A. Many details of the pathogenesis remain uncertain despite years of investigation. The chronic sequelae result from progressive fibrosis due to healing of the acute inflammatory lesions.

Systemic connective tissue and vascular lesions often form the characteristic lesions of rheumatic granulomatosis. The heart and joints are most commonly involved, followed by subcutaneous blood vessels, serous blood vessels and the brain. Heart disease is the most serious. This disease is often repeated in the acute phase of rheumatic fever. After the acute phase, chronic heart damage may remain, forming rheumatic valvular heart disease. Clinically in addition to heart, joint symptoms, it is often accompanied by fever, rash, subcutaneous nodules, chorea and other symptoms and signs. Rheumatism can occur at any age, but often occurs in children aged 5 to 15 years, with a peak age of 6 to 9 years. Rates are roughly equal in men and women. The prevalence of rheumatism varies greatly. Autumn, winter and spring are frequent.

12.4.1　Basic Pathological Changes

Its development is divided into three phases described as follows.

1) **Alterative and exudative phase:** This is the early stage of acute rheumatic fever. Sporadic inflammatory lesions are seen throughout the body, including the synovium, joints, skin, and heart. Focal myxoid degeneration and fibrinoid necrosis of collagen can be seen, surrounded by atypical cells, plasma cells, and monocytes.

2) **Proliferative or granulomatous phase:** It is characterized by the presence of multiple inflammations known as the Ashoff body. The Ashoff body consists of a central region of degenerated, highly eosinophilic extracellular matrix infiltrating lymphocytes, occasional plasma cells, and fully activated macrophages known as Anitschkow cells. The cell has abundant cytoplasm and central nucleus, and its chromatin is arranged in a slender, wavy shape. These activated macrophages can also fuse to form giant cells.

3) **Fibrous phase or healed phase:** Cellulose-like necrotic substances are gradually absorbed, and the rheumatoid cells gradually transform into fibroblasts, producing collagen fibers, rheumatoid body fibrosis, and forming small spindle scars. The course of disease is 4 to 6 months. As a result of the repeated acute attacks of rheumatism, old and new pathological changes coexist in the involved organs. Repeated progression of the disease and fibrotic scar formation can lead to organ dysfunction.

12.4.2　Rheumatic Heart Disease

Rheumatic heart disease (RHD, 风湿性心脏病) may involve the intima, myocardium, and pericardium. These diseases include acute and chronic rheumatic heart diseases. Almost every rheumatic patient has heart inflammation, but the mild inflammation is not easy to detect and may not cause chronic rheumatic heart disease.

12.4.2.1　Rheumatic endocarditis

In the patient with **rheumatic endocarditis** (Fig. 12-7) the mitral valve is mostly attacked, followed by mitral and aortic combined involvement. Aortic, tricuspid valve and pulmonary valve are rarely involved.

1) The myxoid degeneration and fibrinoid necrosis are present in the valve, the serous exudate and inflammatory cells are infiltrated.

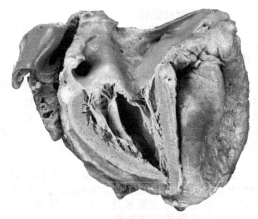

Figure 12-7　Rheumatic endocarditis.

2) The valve surface is arranged into a single row of beads with size of 1–3mm, gray-white, translucent, warty, and it is not easy to fall off.

3) Valvular collagen fibers swell, mucous membrane degenerates and fibrinoid necrosis occurs.

4) The intima focally thickens and the wall thrombus is formed.

12.4.2.2　Rheumatic myocarditis

Rheumatic myocarditis occurs in adults. It is often manifested as focal interstitial myocarditis, which is mainly involved in myocardial mesenchymal connective tissue, especially the connective tissue surrounding small vessels.

12.4.2.3　Rheumatic pericarditis

The rheumatic pericarditis (风湿性心包炎) is characterized with fibrinous or serous exudation. Hydropericardium is a result from serous exudation, while "shaggy heart" or "cor villosum" refers to the fibrinous exudates that are heavily layered on the epicardial surface of the heart. Large amount of fibrinous exudation cannot be absorbed completely leading to organization with consequence of constrictive pericarditis.

12.4.3　Rheumatic Arteritis

In the patient with **rheumatic arteritis** (风湿性动脉炎), any arteries can be involved. The small artery involvement is common, such as coronary artery, renal artery, mesenteric artery, cerebral artery and pulmonary artery, etc. In the acute phase, mucous degeneration, fibrinoid necrosis and lymphocyte infiltration of the vascular wall are prominent and accompanied by formation of Ashoff body. In the late stage, vascular walls are thickened with fibrosis and the vascular cavity becomes narrow accompanied with thrombosis.

12.5　Infective Endocarditis

Infective endocarditis (IE) (感染性心内膜炎) is a serious infection which requires prompt diagnosis and intervention. It is characterized by microbial invasion of heart valves or the mural endocardium. Pathogenic microorganisms are mainly bacteria. The disease can be divided into two types: acute infective endocarditis and subacute infective endocarditis. The former is caused by virulent pathogens and has severe systemic poisoning symptoms. The pathogen of the latter infection is weak, the course is longer, the disease is mild, and the symptoms are mild. Infective endocarditis can be seen at any age and is common in male adults.

12.5.1　Etiology and Pathogenesis

Infection occurs when organisms are implanted on the endocardial surface during episodes of bacteremia. The causative organisms differ depending on the underlying risk factors. The cases with prosthetic heart valves, intravenous drug abuse and some previous cases of endocarditis are caused most commonly by streptococci viridans. The more virulent bacteria common to skin can attack both deformed and healthy valves and is responsible for 10% to 20% of cases overall. In about 10% of cases, no organism can be isolated from the blood. This is attributed to previous antibiotic therapy or difficulties in isolating the offending agent, or because deeply embedded organisms within the enlarging vegetation are not released into the blood.

The disease usually presents as insidious and lasts for weeks to months, and most patients recover with appropriate antibiotic treatment.

12.5.2　Pathological Feature

12.5.2.1　Acute infective endocarditis

Most of the **acute infective endocarditis** (急性感染性心内膜炎) have normal endocardia. It is most common in the mitral or aortic valve while the tricuspid and pulmonary valves are rarely invaded. It leads to incomplete closure of heart valves and blood backflow. Vegetation is grayish yellow or grayish green with soft texture. An embolus with bacteria causes the infarction of certain organs. The tissue necroses at the bottom of the valvular ulcer. A large number of neutrophils are infiltrated, and the vegetation is thrombus, which is mixed with necrotic tissue. The disease progresses rapidly. Despite treatment, more than 50 % of cases die within days or weeks of the original onset. In some cases, a large number of scars are formed due to severe valve failure, resulting in valve closure and/or valve symptomatic treatment.

12.5.2.2　Subacute infective endocarditis (亚急性感染性心内膜炎)

1) Heart: The lesions are mainly involved in mitral and aortic valves. A neoplasm is often formed at the valve or defect of the original lesion. A single or plurality of organisms, large or small in size, form vegetations. The vegetation is composed of platelets, cellulose, necrotic tissue, inflammatory cells and bacterial colonies.

2) **Blood vessel:** The embolization is caused by the disintegration of the vegetations, which causes arterial embolism. Embolism is common in the brain, followed by the kidney, spleen and heart, causing infarction in the corresponding parts.

3) **Kidney:** Due to the long-term release of antigen into blood by pathogenic bacteria, the formation of immune complex can be induced. Most of the cases can cause focal glomerulonephritis. Diffuse glomerulonephritis can occur in a few cases.

4) **Sepsis:** The bacteria and toxins in the growths enter the bloodstream. The patient has a persistent fever. There is bleeding in the skin, mucous membranes and fundus. Anemia can occur in patients.

Summary

心血管系统疾病在我国乃至世界呈现多发趋势，所以了解心血管系统疾的病因、病变特点、临床病理联系是十分重要的。病理医学基础知识中关于心血管系统疾病的重点知识内容总结如下：

一、动脉粥样硬化

好发于大、中动脉；动脉粥样硬化的基本病变：脂纹期、纤维斑块期、粥样斑块期；动脉粥样硬化的病理变化：心脏、脑。

二、原发性高血压

高血压是一种细小动脉(肾入球动脉、视网膜动脉)的长期痉挛；属于血管壁玻璃样变；良性高血压的病理变化：累及心脏、累及肾脏、累及大脑；恶性高血压（急进型高血压）：属于纤维素样坏死。

三、风湿性心脏病

最具特征性的改变：可有Aschoff小体（枭眼细胞）形成；最有诊断意义；风心病主要累及心肌间质；风心病最主要累及二尖瓣；慢性风心病主要累及二尖瓣和主动脉瓣。

四、感染性心内膜炎

急性感染性心内膜炎：单独侵犯二尖瓣或主动脉瓣，三尖瓣和肺动脉瓣很少受累。瓣膜闭锁缘处常形成结节较大的赘生物，赘生物呈灰黄色或灰绿色。亚急性感染性心内膜炎：主要累及二尖瓣和主动脉瓣。常在原有病变的瓣膜或缺损的间隔上形成赘生物。赘生物单个或多个，体积较大或大小不一，呈菜花状、息肉状。

Wu Tian (吴甜)

Part V Cardiovascular Pathophysiology

Chapter 13   Shock

13.1   Etiology and Classification

Many causes can induce **shock** (休克), so it is necessary to classify shock according to its etiology (Table 13-1) and pathogenesis, which helps to take appropriate clinical treatment measures.

13.1.1 According to Causes

Table 13-1   Classification of shock according to causes

Causes	Classification
Loss of blood /fluid	Hemorrhagic/Dehydration shock
Burn	Burn shock
Trauma	Traumatic shock
Infection	Septic shock
Anaphylaxis	Anaphylactic shock
Heart failure	Cardiogenic shock
Dysfunction of nervous system	Neurogenic shock

13.1.2 According to Pathogenesis of Development

Effective perfusion is the foundation of maintaining normal function of life. It consists of three major parts: ① Sufficient blood volume. ② Normal function of vasoconstriction and vasodilation. ③ Normal function of the heart. Various pathogenic factors can alter any of these major determinants and further influence effective perfusion of tissue, finally leading to shock. Accordingly, shock can be classified into three types: **hypovolemic shock, vasogenic shock** and **cardiogenic shock** (Table 13-2).

Table 13-2   Classification of shock according to pathogenesis

Shock type	Factors of effective perfusion	Initial event
Hypovolemic shock	Sufficient blood volume	Decreased
Vasogenic shock	Adequate capacity of vascular bed	Increased
Cardiogenic shock	Normal function of heart pump failure	Impaired

13.2   Pathogenesis of Shock

The specific pathogenesis of shock is not totally clear. The widely recognized cause now includes disturbance of microcirculation and many alterations occurring at cellular and molecular levels.

13.2.1 Microcirculatory Mechanisms

It is widely accepted that shock is mainly a syndrome of microcirculation disturbance. According to the different fluid changes in microcirculation, shock may develop through three general stages: **ischemic hypoxia stage, stagnant hypoxia stage** and **microcirculatory failure stage** (Fig. 13-1).

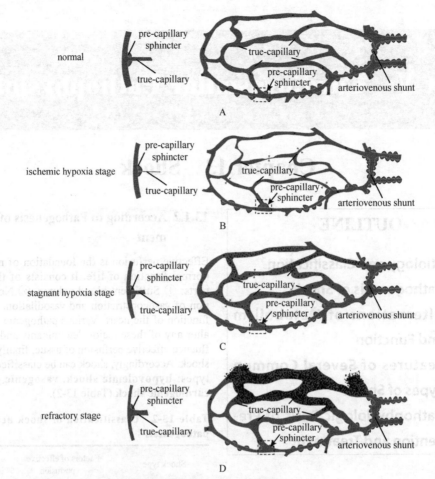

Figure 13-1   Alteration of microcirculation in different stages of shock.

13.2.1.1 Ischemic hypoxia stage (Compensatory Stage)

At this stage, compensatory mechanisms are activated and perfusion of vital organs is maintained.

1) Characteristics of microcirculatory alterations: This stage is the early stage of shock. Persistent peripheral vasoconstriction causes the tissue and cell perfusion decrease gradually. **Sympathetico-adrenomedullary system** (交感-肾上腺髓质系统) is activated, which takes an effect on α-receptors and originates the arterioles and pre-capillary sphincters constriction. In addition, the general activation of sympathetico-adrenomedullary system also leads to **arteriovenous shunt** opening by the effect on β-receptors. Pre-capillary resistance increases and microcirculatory blood flow slows down. Blood mainly flows from micro-arteries to micro-veins through arteriovenous shunts and markedly reduces the tissue perfusion, leading to tissue ischemia and hypoxia. (ischemic hypoxia stage, Fig. 13-1B)

2) Mechanisms of microcirculatory disturbance: The mechanisms include two aspects. Firstly, microcirculation disturbance is mainly caused by the general activation of sympathetic adrenal system. The mechanisms of sympathetic system activation are different according to different types of shock. For example, the vital reason of hypovolemic shock and cardiogenic shock is declined blood pressure caused by dropped cardiac output. For burn and traumatic shock, intensive pain may also induce the sympathetico-adrenomedullary system activation. Secondly, several humoral factors such as angiotensin II (Ang II, 血管紧张素 II), thromboxane A_2 (TXA$_2$, 血栓素 A_2), vasopressin, endothelin, and leukotrienes lead to vasoconstriction, particularly in septic shock.

3) Compensatory significances: Since the effective circulatory blood volume decreases, sympathetic reflexes occur, which can have effect on both heart and blood vessels through the release of epinephrine and norepinephrine. The increased heart rate and cardiac contractility can contribute to maintaining normal cardiac output and blood pressure. Excited sympathetico-adrenomedullary system and decreased renal blood flow induce renin-angiotensin-aldosterone system (RAAS, 肾素-血管紧张素-醛固酮系统) activation, which is also helpful in vasoconstriction and retention of water and sodium. Arteriole constriction and fluid retention may contribute to increasing the peripheral resistance and blood pressure, and finally maintaining blood pressure. While venous constriction may mobilize the stored blood return to the circulation, which can counteract venous return decrease, so we consider it as the first defense line and call it **"autotransfusion"** (自身输血). Besides, as the pre-capillary resistance is elevated, the blood pressure in the capillaries is reduced, which drives fluid shift from the interstitial space to the vascular space. So we consider it as the second defense line against the decrease in venous return and call it **"auto fluid infusion"**. Lastly, α-receptors are highly distributed in skin, abdominal organs, and kidneys, so these organs are sensitive to the sympathetic responses and vessels contraction obviously, which ensure adequate blood flow through the heart and brain.

4) Clinical manifestations: Symptoms and signs in this initial stage are usually directly related to compensatory activity (Fig. 13-2). The patient is usually awake but somewhat anxious. Cutaneous vasoconstriction and local ischemia occur, so the characteristic of skin is coolness and pallor. Blood pressure is maintained even though the cardiac output is decreased. Heart rate is elevated and the difference of pulse pressure is decreased. Urinary output is slightly reduced in response of impaired renal perfusion.

In this stage, compensatory response is important. Eliminating pathogenic factors and restoring blood pressure and blood volume are recommended and necessary. Otherwise, it may develop more serious condition.

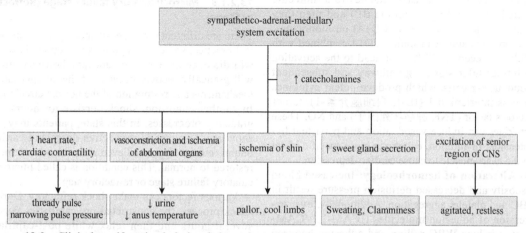

Figure 13-2 Clinical manifestation in ischemic hypoxia stage.

13.2.1.2 Stagnant hypoxia stage (Reversible decompensated stage)

It is a progressive decompensated phase with the characteristic of tissue hypoperfusion, worsening circulatory and metabolic imbalance.

1) Alterations of microcirculation and tissue perfusion: Even though the sympathetic adrenomedullary system stimulation may show compensatory effects in the ischemic hypoxia phase, shock develops into the critical stage if underlying causes are not eliminated. Continuous excitation will lead to the failing of compensatory effects. The constricted vessels begin to dilate. The blood flows through both arteriovenous shunts and true capillaries. Blockade occurs in many capillaries in the circulatory system. Blood flow slows down, which is caused by red blood cell (RBC) aggregation, increased expression of adhesion molecules, white blood cell (WBC) rolling and blocking, platelet aggregation and adhesion, the post-capillary resistance increases, and finally blood stasis and tissue hypoxia occurs (stagnant hypoxia stage, Fig. 13-1C).

2) Mechanisms and effects of microcirculation stasis: As long as the continuous decompensated effects progresses, tissue hypoxia is widespread. Aerobic respiration is replaced by anaerobic glycolysis, which produces excessive lactic acid. The increased metabolic lactic acidosis can reduce the tissue pH levels and cut down the vasomotor response to catecholamines (CAs, 儿茶酚胺类). The constricted arterioles begin to dilate, and blood begins to pool in the microcirculation. Arterial pressure falls to enough low level, coronary blood flow decreases and cannot meet the requirement of myocardium, thereby, this decreases the cardiac output. Endothelial cells develop anoxia injury. As widespread tissue hypoxia occurs, vital organs begin to fail. Such positive feedback can form a vicious cycle, so the shock becomes progressive.

The primary pathologic events causing stasis of microcirculation includes:

(1) Acidosis (酸中毒): Prolonged tissue ischemia and hypoxia during compensatory phase and metabolic disarrangement can lead to metabolic acidosis during shock, which in turn decreases response of SMCs to catecholamines and results in vasodilation.

(2) **Local accumulation of metabolic products**: In decompensated stage, prolonged ischemia, hypoxia and acidosis can increase local accumulation of some metabolic products such as histamine, nitric oxide (NO), adenosine, potassium ions (K^+), Kinin, *etc*. These vasoactive substances may be related to vascular smooth muscle relaxation and gradually increase capillary permeability. Large quantities of fluid begins to transude from capillaries to the tissues, which lowers blood volume and further decreases in the cardiac output, and the shock becomes severe.

(3) **Endotoxin** (内毒素): Endotoxin, namely lipopolysaccharides (**LPSs**, 脂多糖), are released from Gram-negative bacteria cell wall during septic shock. Diminished intestinal blood flow causes enhanced formation and absorption of LPS from gut even in other types of shock. LPS attaches to a molecule named LPS-binding protein (LBP) and then they bind to a specific receptor (CD14) on monocytes, macrophages and neutrophils. CD14 combined with "Toll-like receptor (TLR)" can lead to the activation of intracellular signaling pathway and subsequent mononuclear cells, which produce potent cytokines such as interleukin-1 (IL-1, 白细胞介素-1), tumor necrosis factor (TNF, 肿瘤坏死因子) and NO. These cytokines can induce vasodilation and persistent hypotension. In addition, endotoxin has a specific effect on the heart muscle to cause cardiac depression.

(4) **Alteration of hemorheology**: Increased blood viscosity and decreased perfusion pressure result in RBC and platelet aggregation. Additionally, over expression of adhesion molecules (ICAM-1, VCAM-1, *etc*.) induce WBC rolling and adhesion between WBC and endothelial cells. All of these factors may lower blood flow and result in blockade of the blood capillaries. In addition, activated WBCs release oxygen free radicals and lysosomal enzymes, which will injure capillary endothelial cells, and ultimately injure microcirculation and tissue (Fig. 13-3).

(5) **Effects of humoral factors**: There are several humoral factors produced during different shock stages and also participate in microcirculation disorders. Such as histamine and NO induce vasodilation; endorphin decreases the response of constriction by inhibiting vasomotor center. TNF, IL-1 and LTB$_4$ can induce WBC adhesion, while TXA$_2$ promotes platelet and formation of **microthrombus** (微血栓).

3) **Clinical manifestations:** The obvious features of this stage are blood stasis in microcirculation, decreased cardiac output and blood pressure. Because of the different degrees of cerebral ischemia and hypoxia, the patients usually become dull or are in coma. Decreased renal blood flow always leads to oliguria and anuria, blood stasis in the kidneys always makes the same effects. Stasis in skin results in cyanosis and maculation.

13.2.1.3 Microcirculatory failure stage (Refractory Stage)

There are different outcomes of shock patients in clinical practice, some with hypovolemia or septic shock will die once the condition appears, however others will gradually recover because of the compensatory mechanisms and restoration of the normal circulation. In another condition, shock persists for hours and gradually progresses. In this state, patients may not show any response to vasoactive drugs and cardiac output remains depressed even if the blood volume is restored to normal. This condition is called microcirculatory failure stage or refractory stage.

Various factors can make shock refractory. During shock process, the constricted pre-capillaries persist several hours and then relax while post-capillary venules are still constricted. The blood flow into the capillaries gradually undergoes stasis. Several positive feedback mechanisms are involved in the microcirculatory failure stage. For example, cerebral ischemia and hypoxia inhibit vasomotor and cardiac discharge, so blood pressure decreases, which makes shock more severe. Not only cerebral blood flow

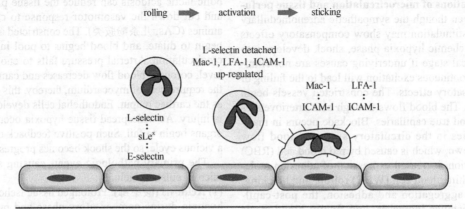

Figure 13-3   Process of WBC adhesion. Mac-1: macrophage differentiation antigen-1.
(CD$_{11b}$/CD$_{18}$), LFA-1: lymphocyte function associated antigen-1 (CD$_{11a}$/CD$_{18}$), ICAM-1: intercellular adhesion molecule-1 (ligand of Mac-1 and LFA-1), sLe^x: sialylated oligosaccharide Lewis^x (ligand of selectin)

but also myocardial blood flow will reduce in severe shock. This will lead to less effective heart function, and finally shock will be worse and worse.

The severe changes in this stage are cardiac depression, failure of vasoconstriction responses, injury of vessels and tissue hypoxia. In this stage, the pivotal processes are disseminated intravascular coagulation (DIC, 弥散性血管内凝血) and multiple organ dysfunction syndrome (MODS, 多器官功能障碍综合征). DIC markedly decreases blood flow. These phenomena can explain why we call this stage refractory and microcirculatory failure stage (Fig. 13-1D).

1) Disseminated intravascular coagulation: The mechanisms of DIC include the reduction of blood flow, the injury of capillary endothelium and clotting pathway activation triggered by tissue factor (TF, 组织因子).

The reasons for the blood flow slowdown include concentrated blood, aggregated RBCs and platelets and increased blood viscosity.

Acidosis severely damages the capillary endothelium.

In traumatic shock, some injured tissue release TF, while in septic shock, bacteria and endotoxin induce the TF release from monocyte and endothelium. In addition, intravascular hemolysis can result in TF release.

2) Multiple organ dysfunction syndromes: Continuous ischemia and hypoxia, metabolic acidosis and release of humoral factors, such as lysosome enzymes, reactive oxygen and so on can cause several vital organs injury. This injury is always irreversible, resulting in MODS.

13.2.2　Cellular and Molecular Mechanisms

Several facts have been demonstrated that primary causes of shock can also damage cells. The injury in cells and molecules may induce and increase microcirculation disorder and vital organs dysfunction. It means that the understanding for shock mechanisms has stepped into cellular and molecular levels.

13.2.2.1　Alterations of cellular metabolism

In the early stage of shock, many etiological causes may affect cellular metabolism. However, in the late stage of shock, cellular metabolism function is depressed severely. Interstitial transport of nutrients is damaged, which results in the decrease of intracellular high-energy phosphate storage. Because of lack of oxygen, mitochondria oxidative phosphorylation and uncoupling function are damaged, so they may be the most apparent causes for decreased ATP production. Several products of metabolism, such as lactate and hydrogen ions may result in local acidosis.

Inactivation of sodium-potassium pump because of insufficient of ATP decreases the membrane potential, so intracellular sodium and water level increase, cells swell and finally cellular metabolism is impaired.

13.2.2.2　Cell injury and apoptosis

There are various factors which can induce cell membrane injury. For instance, hypoxia, acidosis, **hyperkalemia** (高钾血症), reactive oxygen species and humoral factors (TXA_2, LTB_4, *etc.*) are increased during shock process. Because of **sodium-potassium pump** (钠-钾泵) inactivation, the production of ATP decreases, so the transport of sodium and potassium through cell membrane is dysfunctional, which results in intracellular water and sodium accumulation and cell edema. Some organelles also tend to dysfunction: the mitochondria swells, lysosomes release lysozymes and then break, which causes further deterioration.

Inflammatory response is the important pathogenic factor in shock process. The activated inflammatory cells can produce and release various substances that attack the vascular endothelial cells such as cytokines, inflammatory mediators and oxygen free radicals. Except for endothelial cells, they also attack on PMNs, monocytes/macrophages, lymphocytes and parenchymal cells. In such inflammatory response, the outcomes of various cells are denaturation, necrosis and apoptosis. The vascular endothelial cell injury can lead to microvascular permeability elevation and intravascular stasis, which may exacerbate microcirculation disturbances. The decreased tissue perfusion in turn may result in severe cell and tissue/organ injury.

13.2.2.3　Humoral factors

Several factors including hypovolemia and some pathologic conditions cause a marked increase of humoral factors in the microcirculation.

1) Vasoactive amines

① **Catecholamines (CAs):** Catecholamines include dopamine (DA), epinephrine or adrenaline (EP or AD) and norepinephrine or noradrenaline (NE or NA). They are vital forms of CAs in human and very important humoral factors regulating cardiovascular system. DA acts in central nervous system (CNS) by regulating excitability, while EP and NE play a role in peripheral target cells.

The sympathetico-adrenomedullary system during shock causes the release of EP and NE. The response of vasoconstriction, increased myocardial contractility and heart rate are beneficial to restore blood pressure and cardiac output. Persistent and excessive release of CAs can lead to prolonged constriction of arteriolar and pre-capillary sphincter, ultimately, exacerbating tissue ischemia and hypoxia.

② **Histamine and 5-hydroxytryptamine (5-HT):** They are produced by mast cells. Both histamine and 5-hydroxytryptamine induce arterioles and venules relaxation. They play their parts through increasing capillary permeability, leading to plasma exudation and making the blood more viscous. Such alterations promote shock progression.

2) Endothelium-derived vasoactive mediators

① **Nitric oxide (NO)**: NO is synthesized from L-arginine under the effect of nitric oxide synthase (NOS). The vital vasoactive activity of NO is vasodilation. It exerts this effect mainly through activating guanylate cyclase in the smooth muscle to form cyclic guanosine monophosphate (cGMP) from guanosine triphosphate (GTP). Recent research has shown that NO levels are elevated during refractory stage, which induces progressive decline in vascular reactivity.

② **Endothelin (ET)**: ET exerts its effects mainly in cardiovascular system and has strong activity of vasoconstriction. ET levels are very low in the physiologic condition, while they are elevated by ischemia, hypoxia, platelet aggregation and adrenalin. The elevated ET level may be related to tissue injury although the mechanism has not been totally illustrated. The possible mechanisms are promoting vascular spasm, inducing intracellular calcium overload and directly causing myocardial injury.

3) Regulated peptides: Regulated peptides consist of 4–40 peptides members existing mainly in **neuroendocrine system** (神经内分泌系统). The vital function is maintaining homeostasis in physiological condition, while in pathologic process such as shock, they may exacerbate disease progression.

① **Angiotensin** (血管紧张素): When rennin-angiotensin-aldosterone system (RAAS) is activated, the decreased perfusion of the renal cortex stimulates the juxtaglomerular apparatus to release renin. Angiotensin, as a member of renin-angiotensin system, regulates the water and sodium metabolism. Angiotensin can be transformed into angiotensin I (Ang I, 血管紧张素 I) and then into Ang II (Ang II, 血管紧张素 II). The latter stimulates the release of aldosterone, which can induce retention of water and sodium and expand the blood volume.

In addition, local RAS in heart, brain, lung and blood vessels also secretes Ang II and is able to regulate cardiovascular activity. So Ang II exerts compensatory protective effects in early stage but not in the late stage of shock.

② **Vasopressin** (血管升压素): It is a polypeptide also called antidiuretic hormone (ADH, 抗利尿激素) containing 8 amino acid residues. Decreased effective circulatory blood volume and increased plasma crystalloid osmotic pressure can induce vasopressin release. ADH promotes compensatory function in the early stage by its antidiuretic and vasopressor activities.

③ **Kinin** (激肽): The vital member of kinin system is bradykinin (BK), which is transformed from kininogen or kallidin (KD). BK is an inflammatory mediator which can induce arteriole and venule dilation. In addition, it may increase microvascular permeability and induce tissue edema. The final outcomes are plasma exudation and blood stasis in microcirculation.

13.2.2.4 Inflammatory mediator and inflammatory response

Inflammatory response with tissue injury or severe infection may cause systemic inflammatory response syndrome (SIRS, 全身炎症反应综合征). Increased inflammatory cells activation and excessive production of pro-inflammatory mediators can induce vascular endothelial cell injury, edema and dysfunction of oxygen utilization. It has been suggested that inappropriate inflammatory response is involved in MODS and microcirculatory failure stage.

13.3 Alterations of Metabolism and Function

Due to the dysfunction of microcirculation, decreased energy and nutrients, disturbance of neuro-endocrine function, activation of inflammatory cells and inflammatory response in shock progress, all these alterations in metabolism and function are confirmed (Fig. 13-4).

13.3.1 Disorders of Substance Metabolism

There are different kinds of alterations of metabolism in shock, which include decreased oxygen utilization, increased glycolysis, increased catabolism and decreased anabolism of fat in hyperglycemia and glucosuria. Increased blood urea nitrogen (BUN, 血尿素氮) and urinary nitrogen excretion in patients stand for negative nitrogen balance.

13.3.2 Electrolytes and Acid-Base Balance Disturbances

In shock process, cell injury and lack of ATP induce dysfunction of sodium-potassium pump and then cause intracellular sodium and water increase and extracellular potassium decrease, which result in cell swelling and hyperkalemia.

Because of persistent ischemia and hypoxia, mitochondrial dysfunction and glycolysis increase which not only lead to decreased ATP production, but also induce **metabolic acidosis** (代谢性酸中毒). This is due to hydrogen ions and lactate accumulation. In addition, the renal excretion of acid products may aggravate metabolic acidosis.

In the compensatory stage of shock, excessive ventilation may result in $PaCO_2$ decrease and **respiratory alkalosis** (呼吸性碱中毒). However, in the late stage of shock, "**shock lung**" (休克肺) may occur and ventilation function is impaired, leading to **respiratory acidosis** (呼吸性酸中毒).

13.3.3 Organ Dysfunction

Widespread and prolonged tissue ischemia and hypoxia, acidosis and inflammatory response may in-

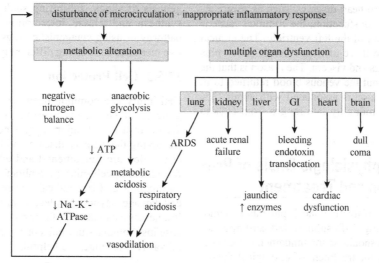

Figure 13-4 Alterations of Metabolism and Function in shock. ↑increased; ↓decreased.
GI: gastrointestinal tract.

duce organ injury and dysfunction. The vital organs, such as heart, brain, lung and gastrointestinal tract are often affected. More than two organs dysfunction occurring in patients without pre-existing organ dysfunction is called multiple organ dysfunction syndrome (MODS). MODS is a severe state which can rapidly deplete compensatory ability. It has been suggested that MODS is the common cause of death in shock.

13.4 Features of Several Common Types of Shock

13.4.1 Hypovolemic Shock

The causes of hypovolemic shock are loss of whole blood (hemorrhage), plasma (burns) and extracellular fluid (vomiting or diarrhea). Therefore, the most apparent character is descending circulatory blood volume. Hypovolemic shock occurs when there is a loss of 15%–20% blood volume.

Hypovolemic shock is the most common type of shock in clinical practice. Researches about its pathogenesis and manifestation are wide. It is worth mentioning that acute renal failure (shock kidney) and endotoxemia induced hemorrhage mechanism is related to ischemia of kidney and gut.

13.4.2 Septic Shock

Septic shock is due to severe infection of mostly gram-negative bacteria with high mortality rate (40%–50%). In addition, virus, rickettsia are usually the causes of septic shock. The outcome of septic shock may be MODS, even when appropriate therapy is performed.

Etiologies trigger defense mechanisms by invading microorganisms or widely by tissue injury inducing septic shock. The direct tissue injury or ischemia/reperfusion injury can cause an elevation of microorganisms and endotoxins from intestinal tract into blood; especially gram-negative bacteria endotoxin and endogenous cytokine have been suggested as initiators and mediators. The pathogenesis of septic shock is related to several mechanisms, such as the release of cytokines, the activation of neutrophils, monocytes and vascular endothelial cells. The activation of the complement system and the fibrinolytic system are also involved in the process. So the pathologic progress that result in the septic shock, are complicated outcomes of microbial products that dysregulate inflammatory mediator release and regulation of several vital pathways.

13.4.3 Anaphylactic Shock

Anaphylactic shock is a vasogenic shock in an allergic condition, in which cardiac output and arterial pressure decrease. It begins with an antigen-antibody reaction, which induce the basophils in the blood and mast cells in the tissues to release histamine or histamine-like substance. Histamine in turn causes venous dilatation, thus causing an increase in vascular capacity. In addition, histamine causes dilatation of the arterioles with a decrease of arterial pressure; furthermore, capillary permeability increases under the effect of histamine with rapid loss of fluid and protein into tissue spaces.

13.4.4 Cardiogenic Shock

When physiological function of heart is damaged, the heart can't pump enough blood, there is inadequate tissue perfusion and cardiogenic shock occurs. It usually results from heart diseases, such as severe arrhythmia, valvular dysfunction; the common cause is extensive infarction of the left ventricle. The clinical manifestations are those of hypovolemic shock plus congestion of lungs and viscera. The reason is that the heart fails to put out the venous blood returned to it. Myocardial infarction is associated with about 10% of cases, and the mortality rate ranges from 60% to 90%.

13.5 Pathophysiologic Basis of Prevention and Treatment

The key progress of treating shock patients is hemodynamic monitoring. Life support and cardiopulmonary resuscitation should be the fundamental management. Apart from the treatment of etiological factors such as hemostasia, anti-infection and acesodyne, there are several essential strategies as follows to correct hemodynamic alterations and improve tissue perfusion.

13.5.1 Improve Microcirculation

13.5.1.1 Volume replacement

The most vital cause of microcirculation disturbance is decreased effective circulatory blood volume. Therefore, administration of whole blood or plasma or appropriate electrolyte solutions in the acute condition is the most effective measure for improving microcirculation. However the infusion speed and fluid volume should be monitored according to central venous pressure (CVP), pulmonary capillary wedge pressure (PCWP) and urine volume.

13.5.1.2 Acidosis correction

Metabolic acidosis by accumulation of products of anaerobic metabolism is an important alteration related with disturbance of microcirculation. In addition, myocardial inhibition, disseminated intravascular coagulation (DIC) formation are all related to metabolic acidosis. Therefore, rectifying metabolic acidosis with alkaline solutions is a basic and effective measure for improving microcirculation.

13.5.1.3 Vasoactive drugs administration

Administration of vasoactive drugs includes vasoconstriction or vasodilatation drugs and must be reasonably used according to different types and stages of shock. Vasoactive drugs must be applied after rectifying acidosis, because acidosis may inhibit the vasomotor response to these drugs.

13.5.2 Blockage of Humoral Factors

There are a number of humoral factors involved in inflammatory response, which is involved in pathogenesis of shock. Inhibiting such humoral factors synthesis and release, interrupting related signaling pathway or using antagonistic drugs have been effective measures for treating different types of shock.

13.5.3 Cell Protection

Cell injury is a common phenomenon in the pathogenesis of shock, as etiology or consequence. Whatever it is, cell injury aggravates shock process. Removing the primary disease and improving microcirculation are fundamental and effective measures for inhibiting cell injury; membrane-stabilizers, energy mixtures and free radical scavengers can mitigate cell damage. Myocyte protection in cardiogenic shock is a necessary treatment, for instance, nicorandil, glucose/insulin/potassium infusions and direct inhibition of Na^+/H^+ exchanger are helpful.

13.5.4 Organ Protection

Organ failure (such as heart, lung, kidney, etc.) is an important cause of death in the late stages of shock. Except general treatment, some special methods should be taken according to different organ failure. **Diuresis** (利尿) and **dialysis** (透析) for shock-related kidney dysfunction, ventilation and oxygen therapy for shock-related lung dysfunction, reducing preload and afterload for heart failure have been demonstrated as effective measures for the late stage of shock.

Summary

休克并不是一种特异性疾病，但是出现在许多潜在的疾病进程当中。休克是机体在各种致病因素的作用下发生的组织微循环有效血液灌流量急剧减少，导致细胞和重要器官功能和代谢障碍、结构损伤的急性全身性危重的病理过程。休克的共同发病基础是组织有效灌流量急剧减少。根据微循环血流变化的特点，可以将休克的发展进程分为三个时期，分别是微循环缺血缺氧期、微循环淤血缺氧期和微循环衰竭期。在微循环缺血缺氧期，微循环表现为"少灌少流，灌少于流"，此期血液重新分布，回心血量增加，对于动脉血压的维持和心、脑的血液供应具有一定的代偿意义。在微循环淤血缺氧期，表现为"多灌少流，灌大于流"，此期发生有效循环血量锐减，血压进行性下降，心、脑血液灌流量减少等失代偿改变。在微循环衰竭期，表现为"不灌不流"，微循环血流停止，可发生DIC和多器官功能障碍等。虽然休克最终会引起低血压，但是休克不能被认为是血压的下降。低血压通常是休克晚期阶段失代偿作用的标志。因此，休克并不一定和低血压有关，同理，低血压也并不一定会造成休克。

Zhao Yu (赵宇)

Chapter 14　Ischemia-Reperfusion Injury

14.1　Etiology

Based on ischemia condition, reperfusion might cause **ischemia-reperfusion injury** (缺血再灌注损伤), it is involved in shock, stroke, myocardial infarction, organ transplantation and percutaneous transluminal coronary angioplasty (PTCA, 经皮腔内冠状动脉成形术) *etc*. But it does not mean all the ischemic tissue cells and organs getting blood reperfusion will have ischemia-reperfusion injury. Several factors can influence the occurrence of this pathological process.

14.1.1　Duration of Ischemia

The reperfusion injury has a relationship with the duration of ischemia. Several animal studies have shown that neither too long nor too short ischemia time will promote the ischemia-reperfusion injury. The reperfusion injury is rare when ischemia period lasts less than 2 minutes or more than 20 minutes. Arrhythmia may occur when the coronary artery occlusion period is 5 to 20 minutes. But this always depends on different animals and organs.

14.1.2　Dependency of Oxygen Supply

As we all know, the vital organs, such as heart and brain are sensitive to the supply of oxygen. In addition, prolonged ischemia can induce the inadequate supply of oxygen, thus, the heart and brain are more susceptive to reperfusion injury.

14.1.3　Condition of Reperfusion

Both animal and clinical studies have demonstrated that the speed of reperfusion and the composition of solution would affect the outcome of reperfusion injury. Slower speed, lower pressure, lower pH and lower concentration of sodium and calcium would alleviate reperfusion injury.

14.2　Pathogenesis of Ischemia-reperfusion Injury

Although the mechanisms of ischemia-reperfusion injury are not totally known to us, it has been suggested that **free radicals** (自由基), **calcium overloading** (钙超载) and **neutrophil activation** play the vital roles in the progress of ischemia-reperfusion injury. In recent years, the relationship between ischemia-reperfusion injury and cell death such as apoptosis has been widely investigated.

14.2.1　Injury of Free Radicals

Free radicals are a group of atoms or molecules that carry an unpaired electron in their outer orbital. There are many species, including oxygen free radicals (OFR, 氧自由基), lipid radicals (L$\cdot$), alkoxy radicals (LO$\cdot$), chlorine radicals (CL$\cdot$) and methyl radicals (CH$_3\cdot$) *etc*. Free radicals are generated in a few amounts during the normal cell metabolism and which are inactivated by endogenous scavenging systems.

14.2.1.1　Generation of free radical

Oxygen free radicals are the most common and important members in ischemia-reperfusion injury. Under normal conditions, approximately 95%–98% of oxygen molecules (O_2) consumed by cells enter into the mitochondrion, where O_2 will be reduced to water (H_2O) by receiving four electrons from the respiration chain. However, the remaining 2%–5% of oxygen receive one electron to form superoxide anion radical ($O_2^{-}\cdot$), or accept two electrons to generate hydrogen peroxide (H_2O_2), thus H_2O_2 can accept another electron to produce hydroxyl radical (OH$\cdot$). H_2O_2 and singlet oxygen ($^1O_2$) are highly reactive although they do not have unpaired electron in their outer orbital. The specific procedure is shown as follows (Fig. 14-1).

Reactive oxygen species (ROS, 活性氧类) consist of oxygen-derived free radicals and nofree radical substances, including $O_2^{-}\cdot$, OH$\cdot$, H_2O_2 and $^1O_2$. ROS has oxidative ability which participates in the electron transport chain and cellular mechanism. Under normal conditions, there are many substances that can eliminate redundant ROS. However, in the patholog-

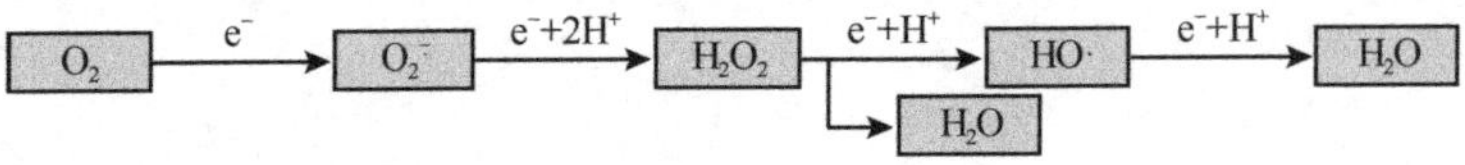

$$O_2 \xrightarrow{e^-} O_2^- \xrightarrow{e^-+2H^+} H_2O_2 \xrightarrow{e^-+H^+} HO\cdot \xrightarrow{e^-+H^+} H_2O$$
$$\searrow H_2O$$

Figure 14-1 Generation pathway of oxygen free radicals.

ical conditions, antioxidative substance is less and ROS is more than it, thus the more ROS can induce the oxidative stress reaction and trigger cell death, such as apoptosis and necrosis. It has been suggested that oxygen free radicals (OFR) in myocardium and blood increases several times at the beginning of reperfusion. Moreover, during the ischemia, the activity and the quantity of oxidases increase. The oxygen radical elevate rapidly after reperfusion, so the OFR will generate to a high level in short period.

1) Xanthine oxidase pathway: There are approximately 10% of xanthine oxidase (XO, 黄嘌呤氧化酶) and 90% of xanthine dehydrogenase (XD, 黄嘌呤脱氢酶) in normal endothelial cells. The activities of calcium-dependent proteases increase in the ischemia duration which makes the transformation from xanthine dehydrogenase to xanthine oxidase. In addition, in the ischemic tissue and cells, ATP is hydrolyzed into ADP and then AMP, adenosine, hypoxanthosine and hypoxanthine. Thus, hypoxanthine will accumulate in the endothelial cells. As much oxygen perfuse into the ischemic tissue during reperfusion, the hypoxanthine is catalyzed to xanthine and then to uric acid by oxygen (Fig. 14-2).

2) Neutrophils pathway: Under the reperfusion circumstance, neutrophils in circulating blood could be activated, which can adhere to endothelial cells. Activated neutrophils can generate lots of oxygen free radicals, which kill pathogenic microorganism by NADPH oxidase or NADH oxidase system. Oxygen

free radicals rapidly increase during the beginning of reperfusion; this is called respiration burst or oxygen burst and then damage to cells and tissue. This phenomenon is important in cytotoxicity.

3) Mitochondria pathway: Mitochondrion is a very important organelle where oxidative phosphorylation happens. During ischemia, **mitochondrial electron transport chain** (线粒体电子传递链) provides primary energy for oxygen free radicals generation. It has been suggested that the triggered reactive oxygen species (ROS) induce mitochondrial permeability transition at the beginning of reperfusion, which leads to alteration of mitochondrial membrane fluidity and rigidity.

Oxygen free radicals not only cause directly the oxidative damage but also mediate a series of reaction in ischemia-reperfusion, including inflammatory factors release, nitric oxide decrease and the expression of adhesion molecules.

14.2.1.2 Alterations induced by oxygen free radicals

Oxygen free radicals are very reactive and can react with a lot of molecules including lipids, proteins, and nucleic acids. The products of interactions molecules are often other free radicals, which are able to react with more molecules, thus a chain reaction is formed.

1) Increased membrane lipid peroxidation: An important outcome of oxygen radicals might be peroxidation of unsaturated lipids of membrane. The in-

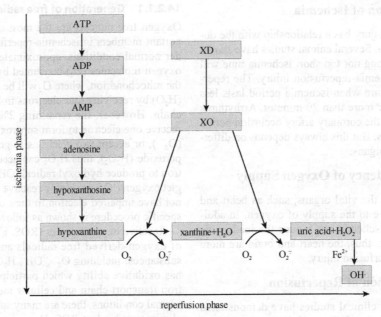

Figure 14-2 Generation of oxygen free radicals induced by xanthine oxidase.

teraction of oxygen free radicals with polyunsaturated fatty acids in the phospholipids of cell membrane can produce the lipid free radical, such as fatty acid radical (L·) and lipid peroxides (LOO·). Oxygen and lipid free radicals are then able to react with surrounding lipids. Alterations of these phospholipids can alter the fluidity and permeability of the membrane, which can destroy transmembrane ion gradients. Lipid peroxidation of membrane can indirectly damage the function of enzymes embedded within the membrane by changing lipid microstructure, which in turn can alter cell function. Lipid hydroperoxides inhibit the reacylation of phospholipids, thus interfering with the repair processes in the cells. These reactions have the potential ability to destroy entire membrane systems, leading to cell death. Lipid peroxidation of membrane can promote the formation of various bioactive substances, such as prostaglandins (PGs, 前列腺素), thromboxane A_2, which can aggravate reperfusion injury.

Free radicals may induce lipid peroxidation of mitochondrial membrane that can damage oxidative phosphorylation and decrease ATP content.

In addition, during lipids peroxidation, free radicals can induce the generation of aldehydes such as malondialdehyde (**MDA**, 丙二醛). Thus, determination of MDA is helpful to indirectly estimate the condition of lipids peroxidation.

2) Protein function inhibition and decreased activity of enzymes of H_2O_2: Various proteins contain thiol groups or disulfide bridges. Oxygen radicals and lipid radicals produced by membrane lipid peroxidation can directly inhibit protein function or destroy protein structure by oxidizing key thiol groups from cysteine residues or by in breaking open disulfide bridges. Amino acid residues oxidation, cytoplasm, and some membrane proteins cross-link to form dimer, which can also damage protein function. Free radicals can affect the activity of signal transduction system by modifying the protein components of the signal transduction pathway or by attacking lipids in the membrane bilayer, thus altering the fluidity and indirectly altering the activity of the signal molecules. Receptor function may be damaged by direct oxidation of the receptors as well as by alterations in neighbouring membrane lipids. Lipid peroxidation may change the mobility of signal molecules and thus affect receptor-G protein-effector coupling.

3) DNA and chromosome disruption: Under the influence of free radicals, especially the interaction of hydroxyl radical with DNA may cause base hydroxylation or single strand breakage, which may lead to cell death.

Therefore, reperfusion promotes the generation of free radicals, in turn, the increased free radicals may aggravate cell injury. They affect each other. Thus, free radicals are a vital pathogenic factor in ischemia-reperfusion injury.

14.2.2 Calcium Overload

Under normal conditions, intracellular calcium is mainly stored in sarcoplasmic reticulum (SR, 肌浆网) and mitochondria. When ischemia-reperfusion injury or oxygen paradox occurs, the concentration of intracellular calcium will increase obviously. This phenomenon of cellular structure and function damage which results from intracellular calcium increasing abnormally is termed "calcium overload". It has been demonstrated that calcium overload mainly occurs in the reperfusion duration. It is caused by increased calcium influx, the mechanisms are not totally clear.

14.2.2.1 Disorders of Na^+/Ca^{2+} exchange

Na^+/Ca^{2+} exchange protein is the main transporter of calcium existing in cell membrane which is triggered by intracellular concentrations of Na^+ and Ca^{2+} for two-way transport. Under normal conditions, the protein transports Na^+ inside and Ca^{2+} outside to form "forward mode", the ratio of Na^+/Ca^{2+} exchange is 3 Na^+ : 1 Ca^{2+}. However, in the ischemia-reperfusion injury or calcium paradox circumstance, the "forward mode" is changed to "reverse mode" because of inhibition of Na^+-K^+-ATPase activity. The higher intracellular Na^+ caused by inactivation of Na^+-K^+-ATPase could activate the Na^+/Ca^{2+} exchange directly and then results in intracellular Ca^{2+} overload. In addition, increased H^+ concentration caused by acidosis during ischemia could activate Na^+/H^+ exchanger and moreover activate Na^+/Ca^{2+} exchange indirectly. Finally intracellular Ca^{2+} elevates. On the other hand, ischemia-reperfusion may lead to the activation of protein kinase C (PKC, 蛋白激酶C), which is another protein activator for Na^+/Ca^{2+} exchange. The activation of PKC is involved in a_1-adrenergic receptor and G protein-phospholipase C (PLC, 磷脂酶C) pathways. Phosphatidylinositol (PI) is hydrolyzed by PLC to two second messengers, inositol 1,4,5-triphosphate (IP_3) and 1,2-diacylglycerol (DAG). IP_3 induces the release of Ca^{2+} from SR, DAG activates PKC further to enhance Na^+/H^+ exchanger. Finally the concentration of intracellular Ca^{2+} increases.

14.2.2.2 Membrane permeability damage

During ischemia-reperfusion, the integrity and permeability of cell membrane are impaired, calcium can enter into the cytosol through damaged cell membrane. However, these damages do not only happen in cell membrane but also in sarcoplasmic reticulum (SR), mitochondria, lysosomes and other membranes. Thus, Ca^{2+} could enter into cytosol and induce cell injury and dysfunction. The high concentration of Ca^{2+} in mitochondria injures respiration chain and energy production. Besides, calcium overload can also cause Ca^{2+}-dependent enzymes activation, such as phospholipase, protease and ATPase.

14.2.3 Neutrophil Activation

Neutrophil are important contributors to reperfusion injury. It has been demonstrated that ischemia-reperfusion injury is often associated with capillary damage and dysfunction which is mediated by leukocytes. It has been reported that in an animal experiment, the coronary artery in dog was occluded for a period of time. In the duration of 5 minutes reperfusion, neutrophil in endocardium increased by 25%. However, some ischemic regions could not be reperfused sufficiently after relieving the occlusion to recover the blood flow. This is called **"no-reflow phenomenon"** (无复流现象). The main pathophysiological basis of no-reflow and microvessels hemorheological changes is neutrophil activation and inflammatory factor release.

Neutrophils adhere to activated endothelial cells and inhibit endothelium-dependent vasodilatation. Moreover, activated neutrophils can release inflammatory factors, including TXA_2, TNFα, leukotrienes and prostaglandins, *etc*. These factors can aggravate local inflammatory reaction and increase the permeability of endothelial cell monolayer, which result in endothelial cells edema, blood flow narrowing and abnormal hemorheology. In the reperfusion conditions, inflammatory mediators can activate endothelial cells in remote organs and induce neutrophil-dependent microvascular injury which is the characteristic of the multiple organ dysfunction syndromes (MODS).

At the same time, activated neutrophils increase the expression of cell adhesion molecules (CAMs, 细胞黏附分子), including the selectins (P-selectin, L-selectin, E-selectin), integrins (CD11/CD18) and immunoglobulin superfamily (ICAM-1, VCAM-1, *etc*.). CAMs family has an important role in the ischemia-reperfusion.

Microvascular damage increases the generation of vasoconstrictor endothelin, and inhibit the formation of vasodilatory substances, mainly endothelium-derived relaxation factor (EDRF, 内皮源性舒张因子) nitric oxide (NO, 一氧化氮), which is a potent vasodilator and the inhibitor of neutrophil and platelet adhesion on the vessel wall. NO is derived from vascular endothelium which plays an important role in inflammatory processes, even cytotoxicity.

14.3 Alterations of Function and Metabolism

14.3.1 Myocardial Ischemia-reperfusion Injury

Heart is a sensitive organ to ischemia due to myocardial ischemia and infarction can cause acute occlusion of the coronary artery. In turn, most myocardial damage leads to ischemia; however, it is known that reperfusion process may aggravate irreversible damage. The vital ischemia-reperfusion injuries in heart include **myocardial stunning** (心肌顿抑), arrhythmias and alterations of myocardium ultrastructure and metabolism.

14.3.1.1 Myocardium stunning

Myocardium stunning means that cardiac contractile function is injured temporarily but reversibly for a period of hours to days after ischemia-reperfusion. It has been demonstrated that in the animal experiments, if coronary artery is occluded for 15min, necrosis or apoptosis would not occur in myocardium. However, the myocardial contractile function could be inhibited continually for 12 hours. The mechanisms of myocardial stunning are involved in oxygen free radicals and calcium overload. The neutrophils activation causing no-flow phenomenon may impair microcirculation and aggravate myocardial dysfunction.

14.3.1.2 Reperfusion arrhythmias

The earliest and most striking electrophysiological response of ischemic myocardium during reperfusion is severe arrhythmia, which is termed as reperfusion arrhythmia. The major manifestations of reperfusion arrhythmias are ventricular tachycardia and fibrillation, even cause sudden death. The occurrence of reperfusion arrhythmias is 50% to 80% in animal trials and clinical thrombolysis therapy. The main etiology of reperfusion arrhythmias is ischemia, which is related to the ischemic degree and the quantity of ischemic myocardium. In addition, the speed of reperfusion and electrolyte disturbances are the factors affecting reperfusion arrhythmias.

The mechanisms involved in reperfusion arrhythmias including oxygen radicals, disturbances in calcium, sodium and potassium homeostasis, and the nonuniformity of action potential duration (APD, 动作电位时程).

14.3.1.3 Influence of reperfusion on myocardium ultrastructure and metabolism

The alterations of myocardium ultrastructure are aggravated after reperfusion. These alterations include cell membrane damage, mitochondria swelling, and enzyme release and cristae fragmentation. In addition, the reperfusion also causes myofibrils breakdown and severe intramyocardial hemorrhage, apoptosis and necrosis.

It is known that energy metabolism mainly reflects in the generation and utilization of ATP in myocardium. Under normal condition, the ischemic injury should relieve after reperfusion recovery. It has been suggested that high-energy phosphates stored in heart do not elevate following reperfusion, instead, deplete further. It means that the ATP generation is lower due to the mitochondria injured by oxygen free radicals and calcium overload.

14.3.2 Cerebral Ischemia-reperfusion Injury

Brain is the most sensitive organ responding to hypoxia and ischemia. It is known to us that ATP totally depletes within 5 minutes in the ischemia, hypoxia condition. Cerebral ischemia-reperfusion injury causes vasogenic or cytotoxic edema and cell in the brain death, such as apoptosis. The mechanisms of cerebral reperfusion injury involve calcium overload, excessive production of oxygen free radicals, inflammatory mediators and so on. During ischemia-reperfusion of neurons, glutamate and aspartate are released. Glutamate can activate the ionophoric N-methyl-D-aspartate (NMDA) receptors and α-amino-3-hydroxy-5-methyl-4-isoxazole-propionate (AMPA) receptors, finally leading to an influx of calcium, sodium and water into cells. These cause formation of cytotoxic edema and massive disruption of ionic homeostasis resulting from the deficiency of energy in the ischemia-reperfusion region. In addition, arachidonic acid and stearic acid contribute to produce the oxygen free radicals. Increased intracellular calcium can activate different kinds of enzymes that cause DNA damage, finally inducing cell apoptosis and necrosis.

14.3.3 Ischemia-reperfusion Injury in Other Organs

It is known that heart and brain are sensitive to ischemia and hypoxia, in addition, ischemia-reperfusion injury also occur in other organs, such as liver and kidney. The process has been demonstrated in various clinical conditions including trauma, hypovolemia and transplantation, *etc*. The Kupffer cells and neutrophils play a primary role in the sinusoidal endothelial cells injury ahead of hepatocytes. Moreover, the activated neutrophils can produce oxygen free radicals and release cytokines to induce microcirculation dysfunction and no-reflow in liver; maybe it can cause hepatic failure.

Besides, ischemia-reperfusion can cause renal failure accompanied by a high morbidity and mortality rate in clinic settings. Under the ischemia-reperfusion condition, renal epithelial cells are injured, which can cause cell degeneration and death, tubulointerstitial damage. Both apoptosis and necrosis occur in kidney caused by ischemia-reperfusion injury.

14.4 Pathophysiologic Basis of Prevention and Treatment

The preventive and therapeutic goals are now focused on various methods such as shortening ischemia time, controlling reperfusion conditions, supplying energy and using some pharmacological agents such as inhibitors of neutrophil, adenosine, calcium antagonists or calcium channel blocker and cell protectors.

14.4.1 Controlling the Reperfusion Conditions

Prevention is the important method to relieve reperfusion injury. To shorten ischemic time, it is necessary to recover the blood flow of ischemic area as soon as possible. It is known that reperfusion with lower pressure, lower flow, lower temperature, lower pH, lower-concentration of sodium and calcium may relieve cell ischemia-reperfusion injury. Reperfusion with lower pressure and lower flow may decrease overproduction of oxygen free radicals and edema in tissue. Lower temperature can inhibit oxygen utilization. Lower pH can inhibit the activities of phospholipases and proteases, which can prevent the reversible and irreversible membrane injury in pH paradox. Reperfusion with lower concentration of sodium and calcium may decrease the concentrations of intercellular sodium and calcium and in turn relieve cell injury.

14.4.2 Antioxidants and Free Radicals Scavengers

How to prevent the production of free radicals and scavenge the free radicals is an important problem to relieve ischemia-reperfusion injury. Now the free radical scavengers are used widely, including enzymes and non-enzyme substances.

The main enzymes that can scavenge the free radicals include superoxide dismutase (SOD, 超氧化物歧化酶), catalase (CAT, 过氧化氢酶) and glutathione peroxidase (GSH-Px, 谷胱甘肽过氧化物酶), they all reduce peroxide to water. The specific process is shown as follows:

$$2O_2^- + 2H^+ \xrightarrow{\text{SOD}} H_2O_2 + O_2$$

$$2H_2O_2 \xrightarrow{\text{CAT}} 2H_2O + O_2$$

$$2H_2O_2 + 2GSH \xrightarrow{\text{GSH-Px}} 2H_2O + O_2$$

Non-enzyme substances include Vitamin C (ascorbic acid), Vitamin E (tocopherol acid), dimethyl sulfoxide (**DMSO**, 二甲基亚砜), β-carotene, *etc*.

14.4.3 Relieve Calcium Overload

Calcium overload is an important mechanism in ischemia-reperfusion injury. Thus, calcium antagonists and calcium channel blockers have been demonstrated to relieve the ischemia-reperfusion injury in animal and clinical trials. These agents can reduce myocardium infarction and the occurrence of arrhythmias. Besides, there are various pharmacological agents used to prevent the calcium overload and relieve the injury. These agents include the inhibitor of Na^+/H^+ or Na^+/Ca^{2+} exchangers, renin-angiotensin system antagonists, adenosine receptor agonists, nitric oxide and related enzymes.

Summary

　　缺血再灌注损伤是指在缺血的基础上，恢复血液灌注，使缺血所致的组织器官损伤进一步加重，甚至发生不可逆性损伤的现象。缺血再灌注损伤的发生取决于缺血时间，组织器官的结构、功能、代谢特点，再灌注的条件等因素。常发生在心、脑、肾、肝、骨骼肌等器官。目前认为缺血再灌注损伤的发生机制主要是自由基损伤、细胞内钙超载、白细胞几个因素互为因果的共同作用。大量自由基引发的细胞损伤是缺血再灌注损伤的重要启动因素；细胞内钙超载是缺血再灌注损伤的原因与结果，也是导致细胞发生凋亡、坏死等不可逆性损伤的主要机制。大量增多、激活的白细胞产生的自由基及各种细胞因子加重了缺血再灌注损伤。缺血再灌注损伤机制的研究，不仅有助于临床新技术，如器官移植的开展，也解释了一些疾病，如休克肾、应激性溃疡等的发病机制。缺血再灌注过程中的自由基也被称为炎症因子，参与了神经退化、动脉粥样硬化和糖尿病等疾病的发生。因此，减轻和抑制缺血再灌注损伤在临床中十分重要。

Zhao Yu (赵宇)

Chapter 15   Heart Failure

OUTLINE

15.1 Etiology

15.2 Classification

15.3 Compensatory Responses

15.4 Pathogenesis of Heart Failure

15.5 Clinical Manifestations

15.6 Pathophysiologic Basis of Prevention and Treatment

15.1   Etiology

Heart failure (心力衰竭) is one of the most common diseases which cause high hospital mortality rates in patients. Its pathophysiologic process is complicated with dysfunction of the heart. There are a number of possible causes (Table 15-1) and in general, heart failure is caused by:

(1) **Decreased myocyte contractility.**

(2) **Inappropriate workloads, such as volume overload or pressure overload.**

(3) **Restricted filling of the heart.**

The specific causes are described as follows.

15.2   Classification

There are a variety of classifications of heart failure, and summarized as follows. Any of these types can occur with another type of heart failure.

15.2.1   Right Versus Left Heart Failure

1) Right Heart Failure (右心衰竭): It is caused by ineffective contraction of the right ventricle. Under acute condition, this type of failure develops into whole failure of the right heart, such as pulmonary embolism and/or right ventricular infarction.

2) Left Heart Failure (左心衰竭): Left-side heart failure indicates that the left ventricle fails to produce adequate stroke volume, thus the cardiac output is decreased. It is usually caused by hypertension, left-ventricular infarction and mitral valve disease. Decreased cardiac output also leads to pulmonary congestion due to increased left ventricular end-diastolic pressure,

Table 15-1   Causes of heart failure

Volume overload
Regurgitant (left to right shunt, mitral or aortic valves incompetence)
High-output states: Anemia, hyperthyroidism

Pressure overload
Systemic hypertension
Pulmonary hypertension
Pulmonary embolism
Chronic obstructive lung disease
Hypoxia-induced pulmonary vasoconstriction
Outflow obstruction: Aortic and pulmonary artery stenosis, asymmetric septal hypertrophy

Loss of muscle
Myocardial infarction from coronary artery disease
Connective tissue disease: systemic lupus erythematosus

Loss of contractility
Poisons: Alcohol, cobalt, lead, disopyramide, amphetamine, doxorubicin
Infections: Viral, bacterial, parasitic, mycotic, rickettsial
Acute rheumatic fever and connective tissue diseases

Restriction of filling
Mitral or/and tricuspid stenosis
Pericardial disease: Constrictive pericarditis, pericardial tamponade, left ventricular hypertrophy, endomyocardial fibrosis
Infiltrative diseases: Amyloidosis

increased left-atrial pressure and increased pulmonary capillary pressure. Acute left heart failure can often induce right heart failure.

15.2.2   Acute Versus Chronic Heart Failure

There are three factors deciding acute or chronic heart failure: Speed of the onset of heart failure, presence or absence of compensatory mechanism and whether fluid accumulates in the interstitial space.

1) Acute Congestive Heart Failure (急性心力衰竭): The characteristic is rapid onset and normovolemic or hypovolemic. Compensatory mechanisms are too late to take effect.

2) Chronic Heart Failure (慢性心力衰竭): In this type of heart failure, symptoms and signs of heart failure develop under the effect of compensatory mechanisms. It can also be aggravated by some factors, for instance, arrhythmia, acute ischemia, infection and work overload.

15.2.3   Low-output Versus High-output Heart Failure

1) Low-output Heart Failure: This type of failure is

caused by myocardial ischemia, hypertension or cardiomyopathy. These can induce insufficient ventricular systolic ejection and result in inadequate blood cardiac output.

2) High-output Heart Failure: High-output heart failure is an uncommon type of failure in clinic. It is often caused by a lot of needs for cardiac output. The function of the heart is normal or supra-normal but it still cannot meet excessive metabolic needs. High-output heart failure is usually caused by fever, severe anemia, hyperthyroidism and pregnancy.

15.3　Compensatory Responses

Compensatory responses are the first response of the body when cardiac output is no longer adequate to meet metabolic needs. The cardiac output may be maintained through these compensatory mechanisms. The main compensatory responses include increased heart rate, the Frank-Starling mechanism, myocardial hypertrophy and myocardial remodeling, the activation of neuro-humoral system can take an effect on sympathetic system, the renin-angiotensin-aldosterone system and natriuretic peptides, *etc*. The adaptive mechanisms are shown as follows.

15.3.1　Cardiac Compensation

15.3.1.1　Increased heart rate and cardiac contractility

The increased heart rate and cardiac contractility occurring rapidly after myocardial dysfunction, induces the elevated level of catecholamines and sympathetic tone. These adaptive responses may be adequate to maintain the whole pumping performance of the heart at relatively normal levels and tend to maintain cardiac output. However, the compensatory response depending on increased heart rate is not effective all the time, after a long time, the tachycardia itself can lead to heart failure.

15.3.1.2　Increasing output via Frank-Starling mechanism

The heart has its intrinsic capability, independent of neural and humoral mechanisms, the increased contraction causes an increase in venous return, but it is discharged by heart itself. This is called **Frank-Star-**

ling mechanism (FS机制). Through this mechanism heart can empty the increased venous return and increase cardiac output. However, the mechanism becomes ineffective when the heart is overfilled to an extent that the myosin filaments are no longer in optimal approximation with the actin filaments, or their interacting sites have slipped away each other.

15.3.1.3　Myocardial hypertrophy

Myocardial hypertrophy (心肌肥大) is an important compensatory mechanism in heart failure. It often occurs in several weeks to months after suffering pressure or volume overload. As myocardial hypertrophy can maintain the cardiac output for several years, it was regarded as the most long-persistent and effective compensatory mechanism in failing heart.

Myocardial hypertrophy includes two types: **concentric hypertrophy** (向心性肥大) and **eccentric hypertrophy** (离心性肥大) (Fig. 15-1). Concentric hypertrophy, the response to pressure overload is associated with increased number of sarcomere arranged in parallel. The wall thickness is increased, which reduces wall tension and cardiac compliance. Eccentric hypertrophy is the response to volume overload, which is characterized by dilation with relative decreased wall thickness. It is caused by increased number of sarcomere arranged in series. The dilation of the chamber results in proportional elevation in stroke volume.

At the early stage of heart failure, heart itself could maintain cardiac output at near-normal level. If there are intrinsic defects in hypertrophic cardiomyocytes, compensatory response would be ineffective and lead to heart failure.

15.3.2　Systemic Compensation

15.3.2.1　Increase in blood volume

Decrease of cardiac output stimulates the sympathetic nervous system, which leads to the occurrence of several events such as activation of the RAAS. Activation of RAAS results in renal retention of water and sodium, so the blood volume increases. Although the exact mechanism of RAAS activation is not very clear, the decrease of cardiac output with heart failure can trigger events as follows: ① renal blood flow decreases, eventually decreasing the glomerular filtration rate (GFR, 肾小球滤过率); ② release of renin

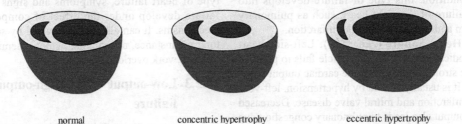

normal　　　　　　concentric hypertrophy　　　　　eccentric hypertrophy

Figure 15-1　Ideograph of two types of myocardial hypertrophy.

from the juxtaglomerular apparatus; ③ renin interacts with angiotensinogen and then produces Ang Ⅰ; ④ conversion of Ang Ⅰ to Ang Ⅱ; ⑤ aldosterone secretion from adrenal glands promotes water and sodium retention. Antidiuretic hormone levels are usually increased in severe heart failure; it can reserve water in collecting ducts. Activation of RAAS, decreased GFR and increased aldosterone and ADH all promote blood volume elevation and increase preload, enhance cardiac output according to Frank-Starling mechanism.

15.3.2.2 Redistribution of blood flow

The stroke volume decreases in heart failure patients, which induces a compensatory response. Peripheral arterial vasoconstriction leads to redistribution of blood flow from skin, abdominal organs, as these organs are less active in metabolism. The blood flows into heart and brain, maintaining the perfusion of important organs. However, persistent redistribution of blood increases afterload and impairs tissue perfusion in vascular beds.

15.3.2.3 Increase of erythrocytes

Because of circulatory hypoxia and redistribution of blood flow in heart failure, hypoperfusion of kidney occurs, which stimulates the synthesis and release of erythropoietin (EPO, 促红细胞生成素). EPO is a growth factor which can regulate erythrocytes production and stimulate the bone marrow. EPO induces the increase of erythrocytes in heart failure, thus erythrocytes carry more oxygen and increase oxygen supply to the tissue.

15.3.2.4 Increased ability of tissues to utilize oxygen

In heart failure, blood flow may slow down, so oxygen supply to tissue decreases. Cells can increase their ability to utilize oxygen by compensatory response when oxygen supply is not enough. When cells are in hypoxic environment, the quantity of mitochondria and their surface area are increased, and the amount and activities of enzymes in the respiratory chain increase. Thus, cells and tissue increase their ability of utilizing oxygen and get more energy supply.

15.3.3 Neurohormonal Compensation

15.3.3.1 Sympathetic nervous system

Activation of the sympathetic nervous system plays an important role in the compensatory mechanism responses to decreased cardiac output in heart failure. As neurohormonal effect in heart leads to systemic vasoconstriction, it induces increased systemic vascular resistance and decreased blood flow to skin and abdominal organs. In most heart failure, cardiac sympathetic tone and catecholamine levels increase in the late stage. The sympathetic nervous system could promote the maintaining perfusion of vital organs, especially heart and brain.

However, increased sympathetic activity causes an increase in vascular resistance and the afterload which the heart must pump. At the same time, excessive sympathetic activation leads to decreased blood flow in many different organs. The afterload of heart increases and tissue perfusion decreases. In addition, persistent sympathetic stimulation may consume myocardial stores of norepinephrine and result in down-regulation of β-adrenergic receptors. The increased levels of catecholamines also contribute to the high risk of sudden death.

15.3.3.2 Renin-angiotensin system

The important effect response to decreased cardiac output in heart failure is a reduction in renal blood flow and glomerular filtration rate, which causes water and sodium retention. Renal function could reflect cardiovascular status in heart failure patients. Under normal circumstance, approximately 25% of the cardiac output flows into the kidneys, however this may decrease to as low as 8% to 10% in patients with heart failure. As renal blood flows, renin secretion by the kidneys increases along with parallel increases in circulating levels of Ang Ⅱ. The increased concentration of Ang Ⅱ causes excessive vasoconstriction and promotes aldosterone production by the adrenal cortex. Aldosterone increases tubular reabsorption of sodium and promotes water retention. Ang Ⅱ also increases the release of ADH, which contributes to vasoconstriction and inhibits water excretion.

Ang Ⅱ serves as a growth factor for both cardiac muscle cells and fibroblasts and contributes to myocardial hypertrophy in heart failure patients. Angiotensin converting enzyme (ACE, 血管紧张素转化酶) inhibitor drugs inhibit the conversion of Ang Ⅰ to Ang Ⅱ, thus serve as a common therapy for heart failure.

15.3.3.3 Atrial natriuretic peptide

Atrial natriuretic peptide (ANP, 心房钠尿肽), also named atriopeptin, is a peptide hormone, which is released from atrial cells. Once the atrial cells in heart suffer from increased stretch and pressure, the ANP will be released. ANP promotes rapid and transient natriuresis, diuresis and regulates loss of potassium. In addition, it can inhibit renin and aldosterone secretion and play the role of an antagonist to Ang Ⅱ. Moreover, ANP can inhibit the release of norepinephrine from presynaptic nerve terminals. ANP level is elevated in adults with CHF, but the mechanism is unknown. It has been suggested that ANP may play the role of a counter-regulatory hormone because of its diuretic and natriuretic action and vascular smooth muscle relaxation.

15.3.3.4 Endothelin

Endothelin (ET-1, 内皮素-1) is a peptide released from arterial and venous endothelial cells. ET-1 is elevated in heart failure patients with vasoconstriction activity. Besides, ET-1 may induce vascular SMCs proliferation and myocardial hypertrophy. It has been suggested that plasma ET-1 level may directly mediate pulmonary hypertension in persons with heart failure.

All these compensatory responses listed above are vital in maintaining cardiac output and tissue perfusion in the early stage of heart failure. However, these mechanisms all have a limited ability and eventually lose their compensatory responses with the loss of contractile force and increased preload/afterload. Moreover, these decompensated responses may produce deleterious effects on cardiac output and result in maladaptive changes in heart failure.

15.4   Pathogenesis of Heart Failure

The pathogenesis of heart failure is complex and many aspects of it are not fully understood yet. There are lots of factors inducing heart failure, such as systolic dysfunction, diastolic dysfunction, altered signal transduction and myocardial hypertrophy. Overall, decreased cardiac output is the fundamental change by any signal or concomitant factor which causes cardiac systolic dysfunction and diastolic dysfunction.

15.4.1 Decreased Myocardial Contractility

Myocardial contractility is the direct source of cardiac output and becomes a crucial factor which affects heart function. There are several factors which determine normal myocardial contractility, including normal quantity and quality of cardiomyocytes, intact heart structure, sufficient energy supply and normal excitation-contraction coupling.

15.4.1.1   Loss of cardiomyocyte

1) Cardiomyocyte necrosis: There are a lot of factors inducing cardiomyocyte necrosis such as ischemia, hypoxia, infection of bacteria and virus. However, the most common factor of cardiomyocyte necrosis is myocardial infarction in clinic. Once tissue infarction occurs, normal cardiac contraction is not maintained. Thus, ventricular systolic and diastolic functions are changed. The symptoms of heart failure would be obvious when the myocardial infarcted region exceeds 20% of left ventricular area. Moreover, when the infarcted region is up to 40%, cardiac shock may happen and sudden death can occur in this condition.

2) Cardiomyocyte apoptosis: Apoptosis plays a vital role in the pathogenesis of heart failure. Cardiomyocyte apoptosis is an important cause of decreased myocardial contractility. Apoptosis is different from necrosis, which is induced by stress such as elevated reactive oxygen species and homeostasis imbalance of intracellular Ca^{2+}. In addition, pressure/volume overload, TNF-α and mitochondrial dysfunction also

act as cardiomyocyte apoptotic inducers.

Apoptosis is different from necrosis, it has been suggested that apoptotic cells initially have decreased cell volume without disruption of the cell membrane. As the apoptotic process continues, cell ultimately dies. Loss of cardiomyocyte increases stress on the remaining other cardiomyocyte. Some factors that stimulate myocyte hypertrophy such as TNF-α could aggravate the process of apoptosis. Another tissue change in heart failure is an elevated level of fibrous tissue in the interstitial spaces of the heart. The activation of fibroblasts and myocyte death result in collagen deposition. In addition, endothelin release leads to interstitial collagen deposition. The elevation of connective tissue increases chamber stiffness and shifts the diastolic pressure-volume curve to the left. At last, gradual dilation of the ventricle is responsible for the heart failure. The activation of collagen could lead to "slippage".

15.4.1.2   Metabolic dysfunction of myocardium

The vital energy consuming process in myocardium is myocardial contraction. Energy production and liberation as well as energy utilization are all related to the metabolic processes of energy in heart failure. Thus, disorders of energy production and liberation may injure myocardial contraction, so does energy utilization.

1) Disorders in energy production and liberation: The generation of myocardial energy mostly depends on aerobic metabolism, which is always impaired by ischemia or hypoxia, decrease of the blood and oxygen supply can decrease the energy liberation, deficiency of ATP results in decrease of myocardial contraction.

2) Disorders in energy utilization: It is known to us, myosin head as an efficient ATPase hydrolyzes ATP and initiates the contraction. However, when the myosin-ATPase is damaged, as seen in hypertrophic myocardium or persistent overload (pressure or volume) even when the ATP level is normal, myosin-ATPase can hardly hydrolyze ATP to provide energy for contraction. The myocardial hypertrophy and prolonged overload are the most common causes of impaired energy utilization.

15.4.1.3   Dysfunction of excitation-contraction coupling

Electrical stimulation and subsequent myocyte contraction are called excitation-contraction coupling (ECC, 兴奋收缩偶联), during this process, Ca^{2+} acts as an electrical signal mediator and a direct activator of myofilaments.

ECC needs an action potential to trigger cardiomyocyte contraction. In the cardiac cycle, an action potential induces cardiomyocyte depolarization and subsequent calcium ions enter into the cell during phase 2 of the action potential through L-type calcium channel which is located on the sarcolemma.

Then, calcium triggers a subsequent calcium release which is stored in the sarcoplasmic reticulum (**SR**, 肌浆网). The release of calcium from SR increases the intracellular calcium level from approximately 10^{-7}–10^{-5}mol/L. Finally, the free calcium ions binds to **troponin-C** (TN-C) which is a part of the complex combined with the thin filaments. Binding of these two substances induces a reasonable change thus troponin-I (**TN-I**, 肌钙蛋白-I) exposes a site on the actin molecule, and this site could bind to the myosin-ATPase and hydrolyze ATP which provides energy.

Actin-myosin complex undergoes a conformational change which is a movement (ratcheting) between the myosin heads and the actin, then the actin and myosin filaments slide past each other and the sarcomere length is shortened. As long as the intracellular calcium concentration remains increased, ratcheting cycles would exist.

At the end of phase 2 of the action potential, the speed of calcium entry into the cell slows down, and intracellular calcium is subsided by an ATP-dependent calcium pump (sarco-endoplasmic reticulum calcium-ATPase, SERCA), therefore, intracellular calcium concentration decreases and unbind from the TN-C. Cytosolic calcium is transported out of the cell through sodium-calcium exchange pump located on the membrane. Decreased intracellular calcium concentration results in a conformational change in the troponin complex and induces inhibition of the actin binding site. At last a new ATP binding to myosin head displaces the ADP and original sarcomere length is restored, thus the diastolic action works and prepares for the next cycle.

In heart failure, release of Ca^{2+} to the contractile apparatus and reuptake of Ca^{2+} by the sarcoplasmic reticulum are all slowed down. Mishandling of Ca^{2+} is the most important cause of contractile dysfunction. It has been suggested that mRNA level of the specialized Ca^{2+} release channels and sarcoplasmic reticulum proteins phospholamban and Ca^{2+}-ATPase are decreased. The dysfunction of Ca^{2+} in the process of excitation-contraction coupling includes three aspects as follows:

1) Decreased influx of extracellular Ca^{2+}: In heart failure, the density and sensitivity of β-adrenergic receptors to catecholamines in the cardiomyocyte gradually decreases, which in turn increases the protein kinase activity and promotes calcium entry into the cell through L-type calcium channel. However, the metabolic substrates which produce energy from fatty acid and lactic acid and ischemia/hypoxia occur in heart failure. In addition, acidosis always occurs. Thus, H^+ can inhibit Ca^{2+} entry inward by suppressing β-adrenergic receptor sensitivity to norepinephrine. On the other hand, K^+ can compete with Ca^{2+} so that hyperkalemia could reduce the cytosolic calcium which decreases the cardiac contractility.

2) Alteration of sarcoplasmic reticulum (SR) han-

dling of calcium: The dysfunction of sarcoplasmic reticulum could reduce uptake of Ca^{2+}. The specific causes include ischemia, hypoxia, inadequate ATP and decreased level of Ca^{2+}-activated ATPase, these all damage the ability of SR uptake of Ca^{2+}. Reduced Ca^{2+} uptake by SR may inhibit Ca^{2+} release for available contractile process. On the other hand, the dysfunction of sarcoplasmic reticulum could reduce reserve of Ca^{2+}. Besides, Na^+/Ca^{2+} exchanger is enhanced which results in Ca^{2+} moving out of myocardium. Thus, the concentration of intracellular Ca^{2+} is decreased, leading to the depletion of SR reserve of Ca^{2+}. Moreover, the contractility of myocardium is decreased. At last, release of Ca^{2+} from SR decreases. The cardiac calcium release channel, called the ryanodine receptor (RyR), plays an important role in cardiac excitation-contraction coupling and the release of Ca^{2+} from SR. While the level of RyR or RyR mRNA decreases in failing heart, the release of Ca^{2+} from SR is blocked.

Decreased Ca^{2+} storage in SR and acidosis are also responsible for reduced release of Ca^{2+} from SR.

3) Dysfunction of Ca^{2+} binding to troponin: Ca^{2+} binding to troponin is an important event for triggering excitation-contraction coupling. Once the Ca^{2+} concentration is reduced or the affinity between Ca^{2+} and TN-C is decreased, the excitation-contraction coupling is impaired. When acidosis happens, excessive H^+ can compete with Ca^{2+} and can combine with troponin more easily; this results in decreased combination of Ca^{2+} with troponin. Moreover, H^+ can increase the affinity between Ca^{2+} and SR leading to decreased release of Ca^{2+} from SR after myocardial depolarization. Decreased release of Ca^{2+} from SR causing inadequate ATP should be responsible for dysfunction of Ca^{2+} binding to troponin.

15.4.2 Diastolic Dysfunction

Relaxation of the myocardium is an important property to maintain cardiac output. As we all know, approximately 30% of the heart failure is caused by diastolic dysfunction. The mechanisms of diastolic dysfunction may be as follows:

1) Decreased ventricular compliance: If ventricular filling (preload) is impaired, it will result in a decrease in stroke volume. Ventricular filling mainly depends on the venous return and the compliance of ventricle during diastole. The diastolic function of the ventricle can be described by compliance curve, named ventricular diastolic pressure-volume curve. If a leftward shift of the curve occurs, it means the reduction of ventricular compliance. There are several causes inducing decrease of ventricular compliance, such as myocardial hypertrophy, myocarditis, edema and fibrosis. However, decreased end-diastolic volume resulting from reduced ventricular compliance may lead to a decrease in stroke volume, low cardiac output and pulmonary hypertension, *etc.*

2) Delayed reposition of Ca²⁺: After each systole, the Ca^{2+} pump and Na^+/Ca^{2+} exchanger empty the cytosol Ca^{2+} out of myocyte and sarcoplasmic reticulum. Thus, the concentration of Ca^{2+} needs to decrease below 10^{-7} mol/L and allow Ca^{2+} to leave its binding sites on the troponin-C. This permits decoupling of actin from myosin and this is a necessary step for complete relaxation of the cardiomyocyte. If this mechanism is damaged, such as due to inadequate ATP supply, severe ischemia/hypoxia induces the relaxation extent to decrease and ventricular filling rate will reduce.

3) Reduced ventricular diastolic potential: The cardiac dilatation will be decreased if systolic function is impaired. Many factors can induce decreased myocardial contractility and decreased ventricular diastolic potential which will lead to the dysfunction of ventricular relaxation. Besides, some coronary artery diseases or systemic hypertension causing coronary blood flow decrease will lead to the decrease of ventricular relaxation ability.

15.4.3 Asynergic Myocardial Contraction and Relaxation

Every part of the heart cooperates to maintain the normal function. If the contraction and relaxation function of the whole heart are asynergic, this may lead to cardiac output decrease. Arrhythmia is the most common cause of asynergic myocardial contraction and relaxation.

15.4.4 Excessive Cardiac Hypertrophy

Cardiac hypertrophy is an adaptable behavior on facing chronic increased volume load and pressure load. Once hemodynamic stresses occur in heart failure, Ang II, TNF-α, norepinephrine and other molecules could induce several proteins synthesis via gene mediator such as *c-fos, c-jun* and *c-myc*. This may induce myocardial hypertrophy.

Ventricular hypertrophy is a physiological response to adapt to increased stress. However, persistent and excessive hypertrophy may lead to pathological changes in the heart and functional degradation and finally heart failure. Excessive myocardial hypertrophy is an independent risk factor of heart failure.

15.5   Clinical Manifestations

15.5.1 Low Cardiac Output

The most obvious hemodynamic change of heart failure is low cardiac output. Decreased output from the left ventricle always leads to limb weakness and fatigue. In acute or severe left heart failure, diminished cardiac output may be insufficient to supply adequate

oxygen to brain, at the same time, patients always present with disturbed behavior, such as anxiety, impairment of memory and insomnia. In the late stage of heart failure, cyanosis often appears which is caused by the circumstances such as low output causing diminished oxygenated blood delivery to peripheral tissues. In addition, peripheral vasoconstriction that causes excessive removal of oxygen from the blood can also lead to cyanosis.

Nocturia means individual has to wake at night one or more times to urinate. When the heart failure patients are upright during the day, the renal perfusion is reduced, but the fluid will be redistributed and reabsorbed in the recumbent position, which results in consequent diuresis. Severe reduction in cardiac output may be accompanied by dysfunction of urine formation via reduced glomerular filtration rate. Further reduction of cardiac output can lead to cardiac shock.

15.5.2 Congestion of Systemic Circulation

In right heart failure patients, right atrial pressure is increased, which is eventually transferred to the systemic veins and result in systemic congestion. The neck vein engorgement, congestion of liver, accumulation of fluid in the systemic venous circulation and increased body weight are the clinical manifestations.

1) Edema (水肿): Edema is a pathologic process, which refers to the presence of excess fluid in the body tissues. In right heart failure patients, edema is a vital manifestation. Peripheral edema probably stimulates juxtacapillary receptors which causes reflex shallow and rapid breathing. Peripheral edema leads to fluid accumulation in the interstitial spaces. The edema initially occurs in dependent regions of the body and is most obvious at the end of the day. Severe failure may be associated with the development of ascites or anasarca (generalized body edema).

2) Systemic venous congestion and hypertension: Systemic venous congestion is the symptom of the right-sided heart failure. Increased jugular venous pressure is noted. In addition, a positive hepatojugular reflux test can be induced. The retention of salt and water causes blood volume elevation, which results in the venous congestion and increased right atrial pressure.

3) Hepatomegaly and hepatic dysfunction: In most of the right heart failure patients, hepatomegaly may appear as the early manifestation. Continuous congestion and hypoxia may lead to hepatocellular necrosis and hepatic dysfunction.

15.5.3 Congestion of Pulmonary Circulation

In the left heart failure, damaged contractility of left ventricle induces left ventricular pressure to increase, and the compliance of the ventricle to decrease, which is transmitted to the left atrium, pulmonary veins and capillaries and finally leads to pulmonary congestion and pulmonary edema.

1) Dyspnea: In the left heart failure, an apparent manifestation is shortness of breath, which results from the congestion of the pulmonary circulation. Perceived shortness of breath is known as **dyspnea** (呼吸困难). Sudden orthopnea is always shortness of breath that occurs when a person is supine. It is because of the gravitational forces inducing fluid accumulation in the lower legs and feet when patients are standing or sitting, however, this phenomenon will disappear when the heart failure patients are supine; gathered fluid is redistributed to an already distended pulmonary circulation. Paroxysmal nocturnal dyspnea (PND) which disrupts sleep is a more apparent manifestation of left heart failure than dyspnea or orthopnea. PND is a sudden dyspnea that occurs at night during sleep which is due to interstitial pulmonary edema. It can be relieved when the persons are aware and sit up. Bronchospasm due to congestion of the bronchial mucosa may cause wheezing and difficulty in breathing. This condition is sometimes referred as cardiac asthma.

2) Pulmonary edema: When left heart function is damaged, cardiac output decreases, and left atrial and left ventricular end-diastolic pressure increases. Congestion occurs in the pulmonary circulation. When the pulmonary capillary filtration pressure is higher than the capillary osmotic pressure, there is a shift of intravascular fluid into the interstitium of the lung and development of pulmonary edema occurs.

15.6   Pathophysiologic Basis of Prevention and Treatment

15.6.1   General Treatment

Different treatments should be adopted according to different causes, such as anemia, arrhythmias and infection *etc.* Patients with hypoxemia require oxygen supply or mechanical ventilation. Decompensated heart failure patients should rest in bed until they completely recover.

15.6.2   Improving Cardiac Functions

Inotropic drugs can slow down the heart rate and increase the force of myocardial contraction. The slowing heart rate is beneficial to increased ventricular filling time, enhanced stroke volume (SV) and increased coronary perfusion. On the other side, if heart failure is caused by diastolic dysfunction, calcium inhibitors may be an effective strategy for promoting myocardial relaxation.

15.6.3   Reducing Afterload and Preload

Once afterload and preload rise, cardiac output decreases and cardiac workload increases, vasodilator agents are usually used to reduce afterload and preload. Sodium nitroprusside is a common arterial and venous vasodilator, which reduces afterload and preload, thus increasing cardiac output. In addition, arterial vasodilator hydralazine decreases peripheral resistance and improves ventricular emptying, so cardiac output increases. In all, using both hydralazine and nitrates can effectively improve survival.

Other vasodilatation agents are angiotensinconverting enzyme inhibitors (ACEIs, 血管紧张素转化酶抑制剂) and Ang Ⅱ receptor inhibitors. ACEI inhibit the conversion of Ang Ⅰ to Ang Ⅱ, and prevent sodium and water retention and vasoconstriction which reduce afterload and increase cardiac output. These two inhibitors have been shown to reduce ventricular hypertrophy.

15.6.4   Controlling Edema

The effective strategy for reducing fluid retention and controlling edema is restriction of salt intake. Diuretics are necessary when the symptoms are uncontrolled after sodium restriction, such as thiazides and sodium-chloride transport inhibitor. In addition, loop diuretics are the most common diuretics, especially in pulmonary edema and severe heart failure. However, there are several treatments for heart failure including surgical therapy (intra-aortic balloon pumping, IABP). IABP may decrease aortic impedance and systolic pressure and reduce afterload.

Summary

心力衰竭是心脏疾病病人发病的最普遍的原因之一。心力衰竭是在各种病因的作用下，由于心肌能量代谢、兴奋收缩偶联以及心脏结构发生变化，造成心肌舒缩功能障碍，心输出量下降。机体为了维持心输出量，激活交感-肾上腺髓质系统、肾素-血管紧张素-醛固酮系统等神经体液系统进行调控，从而启动心率增快、心肌收缩性增强及心室重构等结构和功能的代偿，以维持心输出量。但是长期的代偿会加重心力衰竭，导致心输出量下降，体循环和肺循环淤血。虽然心血管疾病治疗方面有了很大的进展，但仍然面临巨大的挑战。近些年来，无论在城市还是农村，心衰的发病率持续较高。对于心力衰竭的防治应主要延缓心室重构的发生并改善心脏的泵血功能。

Zhao Yu (赵宇)

Part Ⅵ Drugs Affecting the Circulatory System

Chapter 16 Drugs Used in Heart Failure

16.1 General Description

16.1.1 Concept of Heart Failure

Heart failure is a complex, progressive disorder in which the output of the heart is insufficient to meet the needs of the body due to impaired contractility and circulatory congestion. Its main symptoms include dyspnea, fatigue, and fluid retention. Underlying causes of HF include coronary artery disease, myocardial infarction, hypertensive heart disease, valvular heart disease, dilated cardiomyopathy, and congenital heart disease.

16.1.2 Physiologic Compensatory Mechanisms

Sympathetic nervous system and the renin-angiotensin-aldosterone system are chronically activated in the patients with HF. Activation of sympathetic nervous system has certain compensatory effects in the early stages of HF, but in the long term, high concentrations of norepinephrine increases cardiac afterload and myocardial oxygen consumption. This may cause myocardial hypertrophy, arrhythmias, sudden death, and even lead to myocardial cell necrosis directly and deteriorate the disease further.

Elevated angiotensin in HF increases the vascular resistance by contracting the cardiac and peripheral vasculature, which may lead to myocardial ischemia, hypoxia, arrhythmia, and hyperplasia of myocardial and vascular smooth muscle. Increased aldosterone increases cardiac preload due to its effect of water and sodium retention and promotes myocardial fibrosis. The joint actions of RAAS and sympathetic nervous system lead to myocardial and vascular proliferation, hypertrophy, namely the myocardial and vascular remodeling.

Secretion of other endogenous vasoactive substances also changes in HF, for example, increased levels of **arginine vasopressin (AVP**, 精氨酸升压素), **endothelin (ET**, 内皮素) can cause vasoconstriction, and the latter may also cause ventricular remodeling. Myocardial β_1 receptors are down-regulated because of significantly increased catecholamine levels in the blood circulation in HF, which lowers the sensitivity of β-receptor agonist and endogenous catecholamines.

16.1.3 Aim of Pharmacologic Intervention in Heart Failure

To alleviate symptoms, slow disease progression, and improve survival are the aims of pharmacologic intervention in HF.

16.1.4 Classification of Drugs Commonly Used in Heart Failure

Six classes of drugs have been shown to be effective and are listed below along with some drugs commonly used: ① diuretics (利尿药): **hydrochlorothiazide** (氢氯噻嗪), **furosemide** (呋塞米), **spironolactone** (螺内酯). ② inhibitors of the RAAS: **captopril** (卡托普利), **losartan** (氯沙坦). ③ inotropic agents: **digoxin** (地高辛). ④ β-adrenoreceptor antagonists: **carvedilol** (卡维地洛). ⑤ direct vasodilators: **sodium nitroprusside** (硝普钠), **hydralazine** (肼屈嗪).

16.2 Diuretics

Hydrochlorothiazide, furosemide, spironolactone are commonly used diuretics in clinical.

16.2.1 Pharmacological Effects

This section mainly introduces the diuretic effects of diuretics in HF.

1) Promote the sodium, water excretion: Promotion of sodium and water excretion by its diuretic effect reduces left ventricular filling pressure and decreases left ventricular volume and myocardial wall tension (lower oxygen demand).

2) Reduce the cardiac afterload: Due to promotion of the Na^+ secretion, Na^+/Ca^{2+} exchange in vascular SMCs decreases, and this thus leads to reduced intracellular Ca^{2+}, which results in a decline in the tension of the blood vessel walls and peripheral resistance. This reduces the afterload of the heart, increases cardiac output, and relieves the symptoms of cardiac insufficiency.

3) Prevent myocardial remodeling: Elevated aldosterone in HF can cause low blood levels of magnesium and potassium, activation of the sympathetic nervous system and inhibition of parasympathetic nervous system. It as well as angiotensin II plays a synergetic role in myocardial and vascular fibrosis. Spironolactone and **eplerenone** (依普利酮), the aldosterone antagonist diuretics can prevent myocardial remodeling and have the additional benefit of decreasing morbidity and mortality in patients with severe heart failure who are also receiving ACE inhibitors and other standard therapies.

16.2.2 Therapeutic Applications

Diuretics are applicable to mild, moderate and severe patients with HF, especially the patients with high left or right ventricular filling volume or accompanied by edema, or patients with obvious congestion and ecchymosis.

1) Thiazide diuretics: Thiazide diuretics are applicable to mild and moderate HF. Hydrochlorothiazide, one of the commonly-used thiazide diuretics, can be intermittently applied 2–4 times a week.

2) Loop diuretics: Oral administration or intravenous injection of furosemide, bumetanide (布美他尼) and other loop diuretics are applicable respectively for moderate HF and severe HF, especially when acute left cardiac insufficiency, <30mL/min of glomerular filtration rate, or diuretic resistance happen.

3) K^+-sparing diuretics: Aldosterone antagonist K^+-sparing diuretics can be applied as an auxiliary treatment to the severe HF patients with high blood aldosterone. Small doses of spironolactone (20mg/day) can not only reduce the discharge of K^+, but also reduce the outflow of myocardial K^+ to prevent arrhythmia caused by cardiac glycoside poisoning. Combination with other **potassium-depleting diuret-**ics (排钾利尿药) can maintain the balance of K^+ in the body.

Diuretic alone cannot prolong life. It is worth noting that the decrease of blood volume may cause neurohormonal activation, which has unfavorable influence on the prognosis of HF. But diuretics are still indispensable to HF treatment.

16.3 Inhibitors of Renin-Angiotensin System

These are drugs that either interfere with the biosynthesis of angiotensin II, or act as antagonists of angiotensin receptors.

16.3.1 Angiotensin Converting Enzyme Inhibitors (ACEIs)

ACEIs inhibit the enzyme that cleaves angiotensin I to produce the potent vasoconstrictor angiotensin II. Since the early 1980s, ACEIs have begun to be applied to treat hypertension. In recent nearly 10 years, it has been found that ACEIs can reverse myocardial hypertrophy, ventricular remodeling, and inhibit myocardial fibrosis, besides dilating blood vessels. It can not only alleviate symptoms of HF, but also improve prognosis. The use of ACEIs in the treatment of HF has significantly decreased both morbidity and mortality.

They are currently one of the key drugs to block neuroendocrine system and reverse myocardial remodeling in HF.

ACEIs include captopril, **enalapril** (依那普利), **lisinopril** (赖诺普利), **cilazapril** (西拉普利), **benazepril** (贝那普利), **perindopril** (哌林多普利), **ramipril** (雷米普利), **fosinopril** (福辛普利) and so on. They share similar pharmacological effects.

16.3.1.1 Pharmacokinetics

ACEIs cannot be absorbed completely but adequately following oral administration. They should not be taken with food because the latter may decrease its absorption. Except for captopril, ACEIs are pro-drugs that require activation by hydrolys is via hepatic enzymes.

The active moiety of most ACEIs, except for fosinopri are eliminated through kidneys. Plasma half-lives of active compounds range from 2 to 12 hours. The inhibition of ACE may be much longer.

16.3.1.2 Pharmacological effects and mechanisms

1) In the local environment angiotensin II can promote the release of norepinephrine. ACEIs inhibit angiotensin II production and blunts the concentration of catecholamine. These agents dilate blood vessels and counteract elevated peripheral vascular resistance, reduce afterload and blood pressure and increase cardiac output.

2) ACEIs induce natriuresis and reduce sodium and water retention resulting from angiotensin II and al-

dosterone, thereby reducing preload.

3) ACEIs inhibit the production of aldosterone which can lead to ventricular remodeling and myocardial fibrosis, that is, ACEIs prevent or slow the progression of heart failure.

16.3.1.3 Therapeutic applications

1) Patients with all stages of left ventricular failure are suitable for the indications to use ACEIs. Patients with the lowest ejection fraction show the greatest benefit from using ACEIs.

2) ACEIs can be used as a single-agent therapy for patients who manifest mild dyspnea on exertion and do not show signs or symptoms of edema.

3) Depending on the disease severity, ACEIs may be administered in combination with diuretics, β-blockers, digoxin, and aldosterone antagonists. ACEIs improve clinical signs and symptoms in patients who are also receiving thiazides or loop diuretics and/or digoxin.

4) Treatment with ACEIs also reduces the risk of arrhythmic death, myocardial infarction, and stroke. Immediate and longterm ACEI therapy is recommended for maximum benefit after a myocardial infarction.

5) Lower doses of ACEIs are recommended for people with renal impairment because people with renal impairment are at a higher risk of hyperkalaemia.

16.3.1.4 Adverse effects common to all ACEIs

These include a persistent dry cough and, rarely, angioedema (both thought to be due to increased bradykinin levels), postural hypotension, and hyperkalemia. Being toxic to the fetus, ACEIs should not be used in pregnant women.

16.3.1.5 Selected drugs

1) **Captopril:** It is the first and the only sulfur-containing ACEI which is metabolized to disulfide conjugates. It is absorbed from the gastrointestinal tract and the presence of food decreases drug absorption by 30%. Adverse effects produced by captopril include rash, taste disturbance, pruritus, weight loss, and anorexia.

2) **Enalapril:** It is a prodrug that produces active enalaprilat in the liver by de-esterification. It is the first-line drug in the treatment of HF. Diuretics enhance its activity. It may cause some rare but serious adverse effects including blood dyscrasias and aplastic anemia. Renal function may be impaired.

3) **Lisinopril:** It is a long acting ACEI that requires only once-a-day dosing and its bioavailability is not affected by food.

16.3.2 Angiotensin Ⅱ Receptor Blockers

ARBs are non-peptide, orally active compounds that are extremely potent competitive antagonists of the angiotensin Ⅱ type 1 (AT_1) receptor which is responsible for the pressor actions, increasing aldosterone biosynthesis, and the proliferative and fibrotic actions of angiotensin Ⅱ. Several clinical trials have proved

ARBs as effective as ACEIs in decreasing mortality from HF. They are not therapeutically identical, but ARBs are an alternative of ACEIs in those patients who cannot tolerate the latter.

16.3.2.1 Pharmacokinetics

ARBs are orally active and require only once-a-day dosing. They do not undergo first pass hepatic metabolism except for losartan which is converted into an active metabolite by it. All are highly plasma-protein bound with a ratio of greater than 90%. They all but **candesartan** (坎地沙坦) have large volumes of distribution. They and their metabolites are eliminated through urine and feces.

16.3.2.2 Actions on the cardiovascular system

ARBs antagonize AT_1 receptor, thus inhibit its effect on aldosterone biosynthesis, and the proliferative and fibrotic actions of angiotensin Ⅱ.

16.3.2.3 Therapeutic applications

ARBs are used in HF as a substitute for ACEIs in those patients with severe cough or angioedema. All the ARBs are approved for treatment of hypertension due to its blood pressure lowering action, which can reduce the morbidity and mortality of patients with hypertension.

16.3.2.4 Adverse effects

ARBs do not produce cough. Other adverse effects are similar to those of ACEIs.

16.3.2.5 Selected drugs

1) **Valsartan** (缬沙坦): It is an imidazole derivative and prototype drug of ARBs with about 20,000-fold higher affinity for AT_1 receptor than for AT_2 receptor. Valsartan is as effective as captopril in patients with left ventricular dysfunction following a myocardial infarction. Dizziness and hyperkalemia can occur with valsartan.

2) **Other ARBs:** They vary markedly in their relative affinity for AT_1 and AT_2 receptors but have the same mechanism of action and adverse effect profile.

16.4 Inotropic Agents

Inotropic agents are some drugs which can increase cytoplasmic calcium concentration, resulting in enhanced contractility of cardiac muscle, though they act by different mechanisms.

16.4.1 Cardiac Glycosides

Cardiac glycosides are cardenolides that contain a lactone ring and a steroid (aglycone) moiety attached to sugar molecules. The most common cardiac glycosides are digoxin (地高辛) and digitoxin (毛地黄毒苷), the major active ingredients found in digitalis plants, so they are often called digitalis or digitalis glycosides. However, their use overall has diminished due to lack of data proving a reduction in mortality.

16.4.1.1 Pharmacokinetics

Digitalis glycosides vary in pharmacokinetics. Digoxin is mainly eliminated intact by the kidney with a half-life of about 36 hours. Having a low therapeutic index, its dose needs to be adjusted according to creatinine clearance. Digoxin accumulates in muscle, and the volume of distribution is large. Digitoxin is extensively metabolized by the liver and has a much longer half-life so the doses need to be decreased for patients with hepatic disease. It has been replaced by digoxin in the United States.

16.4.1.2 Mechanism of effects

At steady state the Na^+/Ca^{2+}-exchanger extrudes Ca^{2+} from the myocyte in exchange for Na^+ at the end of contraction to lower free cytosolic calcium concentrations and makes cardiac muscle relax. The net movement of ions is decided by the concentration gradient for both ions. Cardiac glycosides inhibit Na^+/K^+-ATPase, resulting in increased intracellular Na^+ and decreased intracellular K^+. Increased Na^+ reduces the normal exchange of intracellular Ca^{2+} for extracellular Na^+ and retains more intracellular Ca^{2+}, so that there is more Ca^{2+}available during the next contraction cycle of the cardiac muscle, thereby increasing cardiac contractility.

16.4.1.3 Pharmacological effects

Cardiac glycosides have both direct effects on the heart and indirect effects mediated by an increase in vagal tone.

1) Cardiac effects: Cardiac glycosides increase systemic vascular resistance and constrict smooth muscles in veins under normal cardiac condition, which may decrease cardiac output. In the failing heart, cardiac glycosides increase stroke volume and increase cardiac output, resulting in decreased blood volume, venous pressure, and end-diastolic volume. Cardiac glycosides improve circulation which decreases sympathetic activity and allows further improvement in cardiac function due to decreased systemic arterial resistance and venous tone. Besides, elimination of Na^+ and water is enhanced because of improved renal blood flow.

2) Neural effects: Cardiac glycosides increase vagal activity, resulting in inhibition of the sinoatrial node and delayed conduction through the atrioventricular node. That is negative chronotropic effect and negative conductivity effect. Negative chronotropic effect is beneficial to relieve the symptoms of cardiac insufficiency. The decreased heart rate can permit a longer period for the heart to rest, and an extended diastole to increase venous blood reflux to ensure increased cardiac output. Meanwhile coronary artery perfusion is improved, which is beneficial to myocardial nutrition supply.

16.4.1.4 Therapeutic applications

Only digoxin is available in the U.S. Digoxin is indicated in patients with severe left ventricular systolic dysfunction, but not in patients with diastolic or right HF. Digoxin is not required for the patients with mild to moderate HF since ACEIs and diuretics can produce good therapeutic effects to them. Due to its vagal activity, digoxin can be applied in HF with atrial fibrillation.

16.4.1.5 Adverse effects, toxicity and interaction

Cardiac glycosides can cause many and even fatal adverse effects due to their narrow therapeutic index, including cardiac effects, gastrointestinal effects and central nervous system effects.

1) Cardiac effects: The common cardiac side effect is arrhythmias, including almost every type of arrhythmia. Receiving thiazides or loop diuretics or other conditions which result in decreased intracellular potassium predispose these side effects. Potassium sparing diuretic or supplementation with potassium chloride can usually prevent it from occurring. Hypercalcemia and hypomagnesemia also predispose digoxin toxicity.

2) Gastrointestinal effects: Cardiac glycosides cause anorexia, nausea, and vomiting through their direct action on gastrointestinal sites or stimulation of the chemoreceptor trigger zone (CTZ).

3) Central nervous system effects: Using cardiac glycosides may result in headache, fatigue, confusion, visual disturbances including blurred vision, alteration of color perception, and halos on dark objects.

4) Treatment: Toxicity is treated primarily by discontinuing the drug. Potassium and **sodium phenytoin** (苯妥英钠) can replace Na^+/K^+-ATPase from cardiac glycosides which is useful to decrease myocardial automaticity to treat tachyarrhythmias while **atropine** (阿托品) is useful to treat bradyarrhythmia and atrioventricular block. **Lidocaine** (利多卡因) may be useful in treating ventricular arrhythmia. Antidigoxin antibodies (digoxin immune F_{ab}) or hemoperfusion is useful in acute toxicity.

5) Interaction: When combined with **quinidine** (奎尼丁), **verapamil** (维拉帕米), and **amiodarone** (胺碘酮), digoxin needs to be applied in a reduced dosage because those drugs displace digoxin from tissue protein-binding sites or compete with digoxin for renal excretion resulting in increase of digoxin in the plasma levels. Hypothyroidism, hypoxia, renal failure, and myocarditis are also predisposing factors for digoxin toxicity. **Cholestyramine** (消胆胺) and **neomycin** (新霉素) can bind to digitalis compounds and interfere with digoxin's therapy. **Phenobarbital** (苯巴比妥) and other drugs that enhance hepatic metabolizing enzymes may lower concentrations of the active drug.

16.4.2 β-Adrenoreceptor Agonists

β-Adrenergic agonists cause positive inotropic effects, vasodilation and improve cardiac performance. Dobutamine (多巴酚丁胺) is a synthetic catecholamine derivative and activates primarily myocardial β_1-adrenoceptors, with less effects on β_2- and α-adrenoceptors and no effects on dopamine receptors. Dobutamine leads to an increase in intracellular cAMP and finally results in activation of slow calcium channels and increase of intracellular calcium ion level, thereby enhancing contraction. Moderate doses of dobutamine do not increase heart rate. Dobutamine must be administrated by intravenous infusion and is primarily used in the treatment of acute HF or severe chronic cardiac failure or is applied as inotropic support after an MI (myocardial infarction) and cardiac surgery. Combined infusion therapy with nitroprusside or nitroglycerin may improve cardiac performance in patients with advanced heart failure. Dobutamine causes tachycardia and hypertension, but it is less arrhythmogenic than **isoproterenol** (异丙肾上腺素). It is the mostcommonly used inotropic agent other than digoxin.

16.4.3 Phosphodiesterase Inhibitors

Phosphodiesterase inhibitors increase the intracellular concentration of cAMP leading to an increase in intracellular calcium and, therefore, cardiac contractility. Inamrinone (氨力农) (formerly amrinone) and milrinone (米力农) are bipyridine derivatives related to the anticholinergic agent **biperiden** (比哌立登) and used in patients who do not respond to digitalis as phosphodiesterase inhibitors. They may produce some symptomatic benefits in patients with refractory HF. They are most effective in individuals with elevated left ventricular filling pressure because of their effects on reducing the pressure and vascular resistance. They are given intravenously only for a short term because long-term therapy may substantially increase the risk of mortality. The transient thrombocytopenia and hypotension are the most common adverse effects they cause. Fever and GI (gastrointestinal) disturbances occur occasionally.

16.5   β-Adrenoreceptor Antagonists

In spite of negative inotropic activity and possible initial exacerbation of symptoms, long term clinical trials demonstrate that patients who receive β-blockers show improved systolic functioning, reversed cardiac remodeling, improved life quality and decreased mortality rate. β-blockers decrease excessive tachycardia and adverse affects of high catecholamine levels and the release of renin which are chronically activated in heart failure patients.

Treatment should be cautiously initiated at low doses and gradually titrated to effective doses based on patient tolerance. It will commonly take several months with an average of three months to obtain obvious improvements including usually a slight rise in ejection fraction, slower heart rate, and reduction in symptoms. Combination of diuretics, ACEIs and di-goxin is necessary to guarantee the effects of β-blockers. It is useful for many HF patients, especially for dilated cardiomyopathy, but is not recommended for patients with acute HF. The patient who also is hypertensive will obtain additional benefit from the β-blockers.

Not all β-blockers have been certified useful, except **carvedilol** (卡维地洛), **metoprolol** (美托洛尔), **bisoprolol** (比索洛尔), and **nebivolol** (奈必洛尔) which have been proved to reduce mortality. Carvedilol is a nonselective β-adrenoreceptor antagonist that also blocks α-adrenoreceptors. Metoprolol and nebivolol are β_1-selective antagonists, whereas bisoprolol is a β_2-selective antagonist.

16.6   Direct Vasodilators

Vasodilators include selective arteriolar dilators (**hydralazine**, 肼屈嗪, *etc.*), venous dilators (**nitrates**, 硝酸盐; **isosorbide dinitrate**, 硝酸异山梨酯, *etc.*), and drugs with nonselective vasodilating effects (**sodium nitroprusside**, 硝普钠, *etc.*). Dilation of venous blood vessels increases venous capacitance to decrease cardiac preload. Arterial dilators reduce arterial resistance and cardiac afterload. The agent should be chosen according to the patients' signs, symptoms and hemodynamic measurements. Venous dilators such as long-acting nitrates will most help patients with dyspnea reducing, filling pressures and the symptoms of pulmonary congestion, whereas an arteriolar dilator such as hydralazine, may help patients with low left ventricular output increasing forward cardiac output. Dilation of both arterioles and veins is required for patients with severe chronic heart failure who usually involve both elevated filling pressures and reduced cardiac output. A fixed combination of isosorbide dinitrate/hydralazine (BiDil) is currently approved for use in African Americans.

Summary

治疗心衰的药物主要包括利尿药（氢氯噻嗪、呋塞米、螺内酯等），肾素血管紧张素醛固酮系统抑制剂（卡托普利、氯沙坦等），正性肌力药（地高辛等），β-肾上腺素受体阻滞剂（卡维地洛等）及直接血管扩张剂（硝普钠、肼屈嗪等）五类药物。其中，血管紧张素转化酶抑制剂、血管紧张素受体阻滞剂、某些β-肾上腺素受体阻滞剂、醛固酮受体阻断剂能够延长慢性心力衰竭患者的寿命，对心脏收缩期功能障碍及舒张期功能障碍都有治疗作用。这些非心脏靶向药物对心衰患者的长期治疗效果强于传统的正性肌力药（强心苷），后者主要用于急性收缩功能障碍为主要特点的心衰，其可减少收缩功能障碍引起的症状。

Wang Yuchun, Ji Hui (王玉春, 纪慧)

Chapter 17 Antiarrhythmic Drugs

OUTLINE

17.1 Cause of Arrhythmia

17.2 Mechanism of Antiarrhythmic Drugs

17.3 Classification of Antiarrhythmic Drugs

17.4 Specific Antiarrhythmic Drugs

17.1 Cause of Arrhythmia

Arrhythmia (心律失常) mainly refers to abnormal cardiac rhythm and frequency. Many factors precipitate or exacerbate arrhythmia: ischemia, hypoxia, acidosis or alkalosis, electrolyte abnormality, excessive catecholamine exposure, autonomic influences and drug toxicity (e.g., digitalis or antiarrhythmic drugs). Both improper impulse formation and improper impulse conduction can cause arrhythmia.

1) Abnormal automaticity (异常自律性): The sinoatrial (SA) node shows the fastest rate of phase 4 automatic depolarization and, therefore, exhibits a higher rate of discharge than that occurring in other pacemaker cells. Thus, the SA node normally sets the pace of myocardial contraction, while other latent pacemakers are depolarized by impulses coming from the SA node. However, if other myocardial cells show enhanced automaticity than the SA node, they may generate competing stimuli, and arrhythmia may arise. Abnormal automaticity may also occur if the myocardial cells are damaged (for example, by hypoxia or potassium imbalance). These cells may remain partially depolarized during diastole and thus reach the firing threshold earlier than normal SA node cells. Abnormal automatic discharges may thus be induced. Increased sympathetic nerve activity, hypokalemia, and mechanical stretch of myocardial cells could increase the slope of phase 4 action potential, leading to the increase of spontaneous depolarization of autonomic cells. Hypoxia and ischemia result in abnormal automaticity of myocardial cells such as ventricular cardiomyocytes; this excitement spreads to the surrounding tissues and may cause arrhythmia.

2) Afterdepolarization (后除极): The myocardial cells produce an early depolarization after an action potential, which is called afterdepolarization. The expansion of afterdepolarization may lead to arrhythmia. Afterdepolarization is a transient depolarization that occurs in phase 2, phase 3 (early afterdepolarization, EAD) or phase 4 (delayed afterdepolarization, DAD) of the cardiac action potential. EAD is thought to contribute to the development of long Q-T syndrome (LQTS, 长Q-T间期综合征). EAD occurs easily when the action potential duration (APD) is excessively prolonged. Factors that prolong APD, such as drugs or extracellular hypokalemia, may induce early depolarization. DAD often occurs when the concentration of intracellular calcium increase. Cardiac glycoside poisoning, myocardial ischemia and elevated extracellular calcium can also induce delayed depolarization.

3) Reentry (折返激动): Reentry is an abnormality of conduction, in which one impulse reenters and excites areas of the heart more than once. Multiple reentry circuits are determined by the varying properties of the cardiac tissue, may meander through the heart in apparently randompaths.

17.2 Mechanism of Antiarrhythmic Drugs

1) Suppress automaticity: Antiarrhythmic drugs reduce abnormal automaticity by reducing the slope of phase 4 action potential, increasing the threshold of action potential, raising the absolute value of resting membrane potential, and prolonging the action potential duration.

2) Reduced afterdepolarization: Intracellular calcium overload can lead to delayed depolarization. Calcium channel blockers prevent phase 0 depolarization by inhibiting intracellular Ca^{2+} overload, subsequently reducing the occurrence of DAD. The prolongation of APD can lead to early depolarization; drugs shortening APD can reduce the occurrence of EAD.

3) Prolonged effective refractory period (ERP): Drugs eliminate the reentry by changing the conductivity or extending ERP. Calcium channel blockers and β-adrenoreceptor antagonists can slow down the conduction of atrioventricular node, thereby eliminating supraventricular tachycardia (SVT, 室上性心律失常) caused by atrioventricular nodal reentry. Sodium channel blockers and potassium channel blockers prolong ERP of fast response cells, whereas calcium channel blockers such as verapamil and potassium channel blockers prolong ERP of slow response cells.

17.3 Classification of Antiarrhythmic Drugs

Antiarrhythmic drugs are divided into four categories according to the main channel and electrophysiological characteristics of drugs: Class I sodium channel blockers, Class II β-adrenoreceptor antagonists, Class III APD prolonging drugs (potassium channel blockers), and Class IV calcium channel blockers. The classification is summarized in Table 17-1.

Table 17-1   The classification, mechanism, antiarrhythmic effects and specific agents of antiarrhythmic drugs

Classification of antiarrhythmic drugs	Mechanism of action	Antiarrhythmic effects	Specific agents
I	sodium channel blockers		
I_A	sodium channel blockers	slow phase 0 depolarization prolong phase 3 repolarization	quinidine, procainamide
I_B	sodium channel blockers	shorten phase 3 repolarization	lidocaine, phenytoin sodium
I_C	sodium channel blockers	markedly slow phase 0 depolarization, marked slowing of conduction	propafenone, flecainide
II	β-adrenoreceptor antagonists	reduce automaticity by inhibiting phase 4 depolarization reduce phase 0 depolarization and slow down the conduction velocity	propranolol
III	potassium channel blockers	prolong phase 3 repolarization	amiodarone
IV	calcium channel blockers	reduce sinus node automaticity, slow down atrioventricular node conduction	diltiazem verapamil

17.4 Specific Antiarrhythmic Drugs

17.4.1 Class I_A Quinidine

17.4.1.1 Pharmacokinetics

Quinidine sulfate is rapidly and almost completely absorbed after oral administration. It undergoes extensive metabolism by the hepatic cytochrome P450 enzymes, forming active metabolites.

17.4.1.2 Pharmacological effects and mechanism

Quinidine blocks fast Na^+ channels, thereby reducing the rate of phase 0 depolarization, prolonging the effective refractory period. It also decreases the slope of phase 4 spontaneous depolarization and inhibits potassium channels. Because of these actions, it slows conduction velocity and increases refractoriness. The drug also prolongs the action potential duration by blockade of several potassium channels.

17.4.1.3 Therapeutic applications

Quinidine is used for a wide variety of arrhythmias, including atrial, AV-junctional, and ventricular tachyarrhythmia. Quinidine is used to maintain sinus rhythm after direct-current cardioversion of atrial flutter or fibrillation and to prevent frequent ventricular tachycardia.

17.4.1.4 Adverse effects

Diarrhea is commonly observed in patients who are treated with quinidine. Hypokalemia caused by diarrhea can aggravate quinidine induced torsades de pointes (TdP, 尖端扭转型室性心动过速). Quinidine has serious cardiac toxicity, which can cause SA and AV block, ventricular tachycardia, or asystole. Large doses of quinidine may induce the symptoms of cinchonism (for example, blurred vision, tinnitus, headache, nausea, vomiting, disorientation, and psychosis). Quinidine also has a mild α-adrenergic blocking action as well as an atropine-like effect. Quinidine can increase the steady-state concentration of digoxin by decreasing digoxin renal clearance.

17.4.2 Class I_A Procainamide

17.4.2.1 Pharmacokinetics

Procainamide is well absorbed following oral administration and has a relatively short half-life of 3–4 hours. Procainamide is acetylated in the liver to **N-acetylprocainamide** (**NAPA**, N-乙酰普鲁卡因胺), which has little effect on the maximum polarization of Purkinje fibers but prolongs the duration of action potential.

17.4.2.2 Pharmacological effects and mechanism

Procainamide shows similar actions to those of quinidine, but has no obvious antagonistic effect to cholinergic and α-adrenergic receptors. Procainamide reduces the myocardial automaticity, slows conduction, and prolongs the action potential duration and effective refractory period of most myocardial cells by binding to open sodium channels.

17.4.2.3　Therapeutic applications

Procainamide is effective in most atrial and ventricular arrhythmias. However, procainamide is not the first choice for treating the persistent ventricular arrhythmia caused by acute myocardial infarction.

17.4.2.4　Adverse effects

Procainamide oral administration causes gastrointestinal reaction. Toxic concentrations of procainamide may cause asystole or induce ventricular arrhythmia. Excessive accumulation of NAPA has been implicated in torsades de pointes during procainamide therapy. NAPA is eliminated via the kidney, thus dosages of procainamide need to be reduced in patients with renal failure. Allergic reaction is also commonly observed and some individuals show a reversible lupus erythematosus-like syndrome during long-term therapy with procainamide.

17.4.3　Class I$_B$ Lidocaine

17.4.3.1　Pharmacokinetics

Lidocaine must be given parenterally because of its extensive first pass elimination. It is metabolized almost entirely by the liver and its half-life is approximately 2 hours.

17.4.3.2　Pharmacological effects and mechanism

Lidocaine blocks both activated and inactivated sodium channels with rapid kinetics, shortens phase 3 repolarization and decreases the duration of action potential. The actions of Class I$_B$ agents are manifested when the myocardial cells are depolarized or firing rapidly. Lidocaine has a strong inhibitory effect on depolarization induced by ischemia or cardiac glycosides poisoning. Lidocaine is particularly useful in treating ventricular arrhythmias. The effect of lidocaine on atrial arrhythmias is weak because of the short duration of action potential and sodium channel inactivation in atrial cardiomyocytes.

17.4.3.3　Therapeutic applications

Lidocaine is mainly used in treating ventricular arrhythmias, especially termination of ventricular tachycardia induced by acute myocardial infarction. Lidocaine does not markedly slow conduction, thus, it has little effect on atrial or AV junction arrhythmias.

17.4.3.4　Adverse effects

The most common adverse effects of lidocaine are neurological symptoms, such as dizziness, drowsiness, paresthesia, and so on. In contrast to quinidine and procainamide, lidocaine has less cardiac toxicity and little effect on autonomic nervous system. **Nystagmus (眼球震颤)** is an early signal of lidocaine poisoning. In patients with heart failure, the distribution volume and clearance rate of lidocaine are decreased. Therefore, both loading and maintenance doses of lidocaine should be reduced in order to avoid accumulation.

17.4.4　Class I$_B$ Phenytoin Sodium and Mexiletine

Actions of Class I$_B$ drugs are similar to lidocaine. Phenytoin sodium is the agent to prevent ventricular arrhythmias induced by cardiac glycoside poisoning. Mexiletine is used for the treatment of ventricular arrhythmias, especially for acute ventricular arrhythmias after myocardial infarction, and it can be administered orally.

17.4.5　Class I$_C$ Propafenone

Propafenone shows actions similar to those of quinidine with weak β-blocking activity. Propafenone is considered as a broad-spectrum antiarrhythmic agent, which slows the conduction of atria, ventricles and Purkinje fibers. Propafenone is approved for the treatment of supraventricular arrhythmias and suppression of life-threatening ventricular arrhythmias. Propafenone may cause bradycardia, congestive heart failure, or other new arrhythmias.

17.4.6　Class II β-Adrenoreceptor Antagonists

Class II agents are used to treat tachyarrhythmia caused by increased sympathetic activity. They are also useful in treating atrial flutter, atrial fibrillation and AV nodal reentrant tachycardia. The basic mechanism for treating arrhythmia is blocking β-adrenergic receptors. β-adrenergic blockers used for antiarrhythmia mainly include propranolol, atenolol and esmolol.

17.4.6.1　Pharmacokinetics

Propranolol (普萘洛尔) is completely absorbed by oral administration, and however, the bioavailability is low, about 30% due to the obvious first pass effect. The plasma concentration of drug reaches to peak about 2 hours after oral administration, but individual differences are large. Propranolol is mainly metabolized in the liver, and excreted by the kidneys. The half-life is obviously prolonged with liver injury.

17.4.6.2　Pharmacological effects and mechanism

β-adrenoreceptor antagonists reduce phase 4 depolarization, depress automaticity, prolong AV conduction, and decrease heart rate and myocardial contractility.

17.4.6.3　Therapeutic applications

Propranolol is mainly used to treat rapid supraventricular arrhythmias, especially in the treatment of sinus tachycardia caused by high sympathetic excitability, hyperthyroidism, and adrenal pheochromocytoma.

17.4.6.4   Adverse effects

Propranolol, a nonselective β-adrenoceptor antagonist, can cause sinus bradycardia, atrioventricular block, hypotension, depression, memory loss, myocardial depression, and bronchospasm. Long-term application of propranolol may induce abnormal metabolism of lipids and glucose, so patients with hyperglycemia and hyperlipidemia should use cautiously.

1) Atenolol (阿替洛尔): Atenolol is a long-acting selective β₁-adrenoceptor antagonist which can be used orally. The action of Atenolol is similar to that of propranolol. Because of the strong selectivity to the heart, atenolol can be used in patients with diabetes and asthma, but the dose should not be too high.

2) Esmolol (艾司洛尔): Esmolol selectively blocks β₁-adrenoceptor. The effect is extremely short. Esmolol is used to treat ventricular arrhythmia and administered by infusion.

17.4.7   Class Ⅲ Potassium Channel Blockers

Class Ⅲ agents prolong the action potential duration and effective refractory period of myocardial cells. These drugs act by interfering with outward K^+ currents or inward Na^+ currents.

Amiodarone: Amiodarone contains iodine and its structure is similar to thyroxine. Amiodarone has a wide range of pharmacological effects. The antiarrhythmic effect and its toxicity are related to its action on nuclear thyroid hormone receptors.

17.4.7.1   Pharmacokinetics

Amiodarone has high lipid solubility and can be administered orally or intravenously. The bioavailability of aminodarone varies from 35% to 65% depending on the individual. Amiodarone undergoes hepatic metabolism. Its main metabolite desethylamiodarone remains biological activity, prolonging the half-life of amiodarone to several weeks. Amiodarone distributes extensively in adipose tissue.

17.4.7.2   Pharmacological effects and mechanism

Amiodarone blocks K^+ channels, diminishes the outward potassium current during repolarization of myocardial cells, thus, prolongs phase 3 of APD and ERP.

17.4.7.3   Therapeutic applications

Amiodarone is a broad-spectrum antiarrhythmic drug. It is effective in the treatment of atrial flutter, atrial fibrillation, supraventricular tachycardia and ventricular tachycardia.

17.4.7.4   Adverse effects

All Class Ⅲ drugs have the potential to induce arrhythmias. Cardiac toxicities include sinus bradycardia, atrioventricular block, Q-T interval prolongation and the tip torsion ventricular tachycardia. Amiodarone produces dose-related and cumulative adverse effects especially gastrointestinal (GI) related effects. Other noncardiac adverse effects include pulmonary fibrosis, interstitial pneumonia, hyper- or hypothyroxinemia, hepatotoxicity, photosensitivity and corneal microdeposits precipitation. Pulmonary function and serum T_3, T_4 levels should be monitored regularly during therapy with amiodarone.

17.4.8   Class Ⅳ Calcium Channel Blockers

Class Ⅳ antiarrhythmic drugs are calcium channel blockers. They inhibit both activation and inactivation of L-type calcium channels. Verapamil is commonly used to treat supraventricular arrhythmia.

17.4.8.1   Pharmacokinetics

Verapamil is absorbed completely and rapidly after oral administration, while the oral bioavailability of verapamil is low due to the obvious first pass elimination. Verapamil undergoes hepatic metabolism, thus, it should be administered cautiously to patients with hepatic dysfunction.

17.4.8.2   Pharmacological effects and mechanism

Verapamil selectively blocks L-type calcium channel. It inhibits the calcium influx dependent phase 4 depolarization of AV node. Verapamil decreases the automaticity of SA node, inhibits the abnormal automaticity of atria, ventricle and Purkinje fibers during ischemia, thus reducing or eliminating the triggered activity caused by afterdepolarization. Verapamil depresses AV node conduction, terminates the reentry of AV node, thus, slows ventricular rate in atrial flutter and atrial fibrillation. Verapamil also increases the effective refractory period of the SA node and AV node.

17.4.8.3   Therapeutic applications

Verapamil is useful in reentrant supraventricular tachycardia, and it can also reduce ventricular rate in atrial flutter and fibrillation.

17.4.8.4   Adverse effects

Verapamil has negative inotropic properties and, may lead to sinus bradycardia, transient asystole, and other arrthythmias. Therefore, verapamil is contraindicated in patients with previous cardiac dysfunction. Verapamil should be used cautiously in elderly patients and patients with renal injury. Other noncardiac adverse effects include constipation, abdominal distension, diarrhea, headache and itching.

Summary

　　心律失常的发生机制有折返、自律性升高及后除级，其中折返是引发心律失常的主要原因。药物通过消除折返，降低自律性，减少后除级，发挥抗心律失常作用。常用的抗心律失常药物分为四类：① Ⅰ类钠通道阻滞药，又分为 I_A 类适度阻滞钠通道，降低动作电位0期上升速率，不同程度抑制心肌细胞膜 K^+、Ca^{2+} 通透性，延长复极过程，且以延长有效不应期更为显著，本类药有奎尼丁、普鲁卡因胺等；I_B类轻度阻滞钠通道，轻度降低动作电位0期上升速率，降低自律性，缩短或不影响动作电位时程，本类药有利多卡因、苯妥英钠、美西律等；I_C类明显阻滞钠通道，显著降低动作电位0期上升速率和幅度，减慢传导性的作用最为明显，本类药有普罗帕酮等。②Ⅱ类β受体阻断药，阻断心肌β受体，表现为减慢4期舒张期除极速率而降低自律性，降低动作电位0期上升速率而减慢传导性，代表药有普萘洛尔等。③Ⅲ

类延长动作电位时程药，抑制多种钾电流，延长动作电位时程和有效不应期，但对动作电位幅度和去极化速率影响很小，代表药有胺碘酮等。④Ⅳ类钙通道阻滞药，抑制Ca^{2+}内流，降低窦房结自律性，减慢房室传导性，代表药物有维拉帕米和地尔硫䓬。

Yang Hongyan (杨宏艳)

Chapter 18 Antianginal Drugs

18.1 General Description

Angina pectoris is the most common symptom of coronary atherosclerotic heart disease. It is caused by atherosclerotic plaque formation or atheromatous obstruction followed by arterial spasm. The blood flow of coronary is insufficient to meet the oxygen demands of the myocardium, leading to temporary ischemia and anoxia. Angina pectoris is characterized by sudden, severe, pressing chest pain radiating to the neck, jaw, back and arms. These transient episodes (less than 15 minutes) of myocardial ischemia do not cause cellular death as occurring in myocardial infarction. However, chronic ischemia will lead to deterioration of cardiac function, subsequently leading to heart failure, arrhythmia, and even death. Angina pectoris includes three types: exertional angina pectoris, spontanecus angina and mixed pattern of angina. Exertional angina pectoris, known as classic angina, occurs when the demand for oxygen exceeds oxygen supply, usually because of diminished coronary blood flow. Spontanecus angina results from reversible coronary vasospasm that decreases oxygen supply. It occurs at rest and is also called vasospastic angina. All types of angina pectoris are caused by varying combinations of increased myocardial demand and decreased myocardial perfusion.

The demand and supply of oxygen in normal myocardium keep a balance. Myocardial oxygen demand is determined by cardiac contractility, heart rate and ventricular wall tension. The greater the ventricular wall tension, the more oxygen consumption of the myocardium. Increased myocardial contractility and rapid heart rate will increase myocardial oxygen consumption. Myocardial oxygen supply is determined by arteriovenous oxygen partial pressure difference and coronary blood flow. When the demand of the myocardium for oxygen exceeds the available supply, the myocardium becomes ischemic. As a result, angina pectoris occurs. Pharmacological therapy is directed towards restoring a balance between myocardial oxygen supply and oxygen demand. The general approach to treating angina is to increase the myocardial oxygen supply through enhancing the blood flow of coronary; or decrease the workload of the heart, thereby reducing the oxygen demand. There are three main medicine categories applicable: nitrates vasodilators, β-adrenoreceptor antagonists and calcium channel blockers.

18.2 Nitrate Esters

Nitrate esters include **nitroglycerin** (硝酸甘油), **isosorbide dinitrate** (硝酸异山梨酯), **isosorbide mononitrate** (单硝酸异山梨酯) and **pentaerythritol tetranitrate** (戊四硝酯). Nitroglycerin is the most popular drug to treat angina pectoris. The effective chemical structure is the same as that of simple nitric and nitrous acid esters of glycerol even though the volatility is different. These compounds cause a rapid reduction in myocardial oxygen demand, followed by a rapid relief of symptoms. They are effective in stable and unstable angina as well as in variant angina pectoris.

18.2.1 Pharmacokinetics

Because of the influence of the first pass effect, the oral bioavailability of nitroglycerin is only 8%, so it is not suitable for oral administration. Due to its high lipid solubility, sublingual administration is easily absorbed through the oral mucosa, reaches the peak plasma concentration quickly. The effect of nitroglycerin occurs 1–2min after administration and lasts for 20–30min; the half-life is 2–4min. Nitroglycerin can also be absorbed through the skin. Nitroglycerin has a sustainable longer effective concentration with 2% nitroglycerin ointment smear in the forearm skin or mask stick to the skin in the chest before sleep. Nitroglycerin is converted into dinitrate metabolites with high water solubility by glutathione-organic nitrate reductase in the liver, small amounts of acid metabolites and inorganic nitrite, which are finally conjugated with glucuronic acid and excreted by kidneys. Dinitrate metabolites have a weak vasodilator effect, only about 1/10 of nitroglycerin.

18.2.2 Pharmacological Effects

The basic effect of nitroglycerin is to act directly on the vascular smooth muscle, especially the venous smooth muscle, causing relaxation.

1) Relax the vascular smooth muscle, reduce the preload and afterload of heart, and thus reduce cardiac oxygen consumption: Nitroglycerin acts on both arterial and venous vasculature to reduce the workload of the heart. Nitroglycerin relaxes the veins in a low dose, decreasing venous return, reducing ventricular filling (known as preload of heart). Nitroglycerin dilates arteries at a high dose, diminishing the peripheral resistance that the ventricles must overcome to eject blood into the circulation (known as afterload). Then the heart works less and the cardiac oxygen consumption is decreased. Nitroglycerin also dilates coronary artery directly to remove spasm and provides an increased blood supply to the heart.

2) Redistribute the coronary blood flow, and increase the oxygen supply to ischemic regions: Nitroglycerin dilates the pericardial vessels, the delivery vessels and collateral vessels selectively, especially in the coronary spasm. The vasodilation of nitroglycerin on the diastolic blood vessels is weak. When the coronary arteries become narrow due to atherosclerosis or spasm, the resistance vessels in the ischemic area are diastolic due to hypoxia and accumulation of metabolites. In this way, the resistance of non-ischemic zone is greater than that of the ischemic area. After taking the drug, blood will flow from the delivery vessels through collateral vessels to the ischemic region due to the pressure difference, thereby increasing the blood supply in the ischemic area.

3) Decrease left ventricular filling pressure, increase endocardial blood supply, and improve the left ventricular compliance: The coronary arteries pass vertically through the myocardium and distribute in the endocardium like a reticulum from the epicardium through the ventricular wall. Therefore, the blood flow in the endocardium is susceptible to ventricular wall muscle tension and intraventricular pressure. During angina pectoris attack, the left ventricular end-diastolic pressure (LVEDP, 左室舒张末压) is increased due to the ischemia and hypoxia of the myocardial tissue, which decreases the pressure difference between epicardial and endocardial blood flow, making the subendocardial ischemia more serious. Nitroglycerin dilates the veins, reduces the volume of blood to the heart, and reduces the intracardiac pressure in the heart. Nitroglycerin also dilates the arteries and reduces the tension of the ventricular wall thus increasing the effective perfusion pressure from the epicardium to the endocardium, and facilitating blood flow from the epicardium to the endocardial ischemic area.

4) Protect myocardium against ischemic injury: Nitric oxide released from nitroglycerin promotes endogenous PGI_2, **calcitonin gene-related peptide (CGRP, 降钙素基因相关肽)** production and release, which protect the myocardium from ischemic injury.

5) Inhibit platelet aggregation: Nitric oxide released from nitroglycerin activates **guanylate cyclase (GC, 鸟苷酸环化酶)** in platelets. The increase of **cyclic guanosine monophosphate (cGMP, 环磷酸鸟苷)** results in a decrease in platelet aggregation.

18.2.3 Mechanism of Vasodilatation

Nitrite ions in nitrate esters release nitric oxide by glutathione transferase, which activates GC, and increases the level of cGMP. cGMP activates cGMP-dependent kinases, decreases the intracellular calcium concentration, ultimately leading to dephosphorylation of myosin light chain and relaxation of the vascular smooth muscle.

18.2.4 Therapeutic Applications

1) Angina pectoris: Sublingual nitroglycerin is the most common treatment for all kinds of angina. Medications can also prevent the onset of a possible attack. Continuous infusion or slowly absorbed preparations of nitroglycerin (including the transdermal patches) or derivatives with longer half-lives have been used for unstable angina.

2) Chronic heart failure: Nitroglycerin can be used for the treatment of heart failure due to the reduction of cardiac preload and afterload.

3) Acute respiratory failure and pulmonary hypertension: Nitroglycerin can relax pulmonary vessels, reduce pulmonary vascular resistance, improve pulmonary ventilation, and is useful for the treatment of acute respiratory failure and pulmonary hypertension.

18.2.5 Adverse Effects and Tolerance

1) Adverse effects: Common side effects associated with the vasodilators result from excessive vasodilation, which can lead to orthostatic hypotension, reflex tachycardia, hypotension, facial flushing, syncope and throbbing headache, the latter due to cerebral vasodilation.

2) Tolerance: Continuous exposure may lead to tolerance. This is related to exhausting supplies of the sulfydryl-dependent catalyst. Tolerance can be overcome by providing intermittent treatment, either in response to an acute attack or by taking preventive measures before exposure to a known trigger. In the case of transdermal administration, therapeutic activity is restored if treatment is withheld for a short period of 8 to 12 hours in every 24 hours. This break in treatment allows replenishment of the sulfydryl-dependent catalyst. Large doses produce methemoglobinemia and cyanosis.

18.3 β-Adrenoreceptor Antagonists

This class of drugs is numerous, and pharmacological effects and clinical applications of this class are extensive. The most commonly used in clinical practice are propranolol, metoprolol and atenolol. In this chapter, we briefly introduce its action on angina pectoris. β-adrenoreceptor antagonists are used prophylactically to reduce the severity and frequency of acute angina attacks and decrease the requirements for glyceryl trinitrate. β-adrenergic receptor blockers reduce the incidence angina pectoris in patients, improve ischemic characteristics of ECG, increase exercise tolerance, reduce myocardial oxygen consumption, improve the metabolism of ischemic area and reduce the infarct size of myocardium.

18.3.1 Antianginal Effects and Mechanisms

1) Reduce the myocardial oxygen consumption: When angina pectoris occurs, the levels of catecholamine in myocardium and blood are increased significantly, activating β-adrenergic receptors, enhancing myocardial contractility, constricting blood vessels, increasing heart rate and left ventricular afterload, thereby increasing myocardial oxygen consumption. At the same time, ventricular diastole is relatively shortened due to accelerated heart rate and the coronary blood flow is reduced, aggravating myocardial hypoxia. β-blockers reduce cardiac workload by reducing heart rate, blood pressure and contractility. β-receptor blockers prevent sympathetic stimulation of the heart. These results decrease myocardial oxygen requirements.

2) Improve the blood supply of myocardial ischemia: The coronary artery is constricted after β-receptor blockade, especially in the non-ischemic area. Therefore, the increase in the pressure difference between the non-ischemic and ischemic area allows blood flow to the compensatory dilated ischemic area, which increases the blood flow in the ischemic area. Secondly, due to the slower heart rate, diastole is prolonged, which is conducive to the flow of blood from the epicardial blood vessels to the ischemic areas of the heart. In addition, β-blockers can increase collateral circulation and increase the amount of blood perfusion in ischemic areas.

3) Influence on the metabolism of lipid and glucose: β-blockers inhibit the activity of lipolytic enzymes and reduce the content of free fatty acids by inhibiting β-adrenergic receptor. β-blockers improve glucose metabolism by increasing glucose uptake and utilization in myocardial ischemic area to reduce oxygen consumption. β-blockers also promote the dissociation of oxygenated hemoglobin to increase the oxygen supply.

18.3.2 Therapeutic Applications

β-blockers reduce the frequency and severity of angina attacks. β-blockers can be used to treat exertional angina pectoris. β1-blockers are relatively selective to the heart and cause fewer side effects than non-selective agents. β-blockers are usually used with nitrates

to increase exercise duration and tolerance in patients with classic angina (exertional angina pectoris). Combined therapy with nitrates is often preferred in the treatment of angina pectoris because of the decreased adverse effects of both agents. β-blockers are ineffective against and should not be used in vasospastic angina.

18.3.3 Adverse Effects and Announcements

Common adverse effects include bradycardia, dizziness, gastrointestinal disturbances and atrioventricular block. Cessation of therapy should occur slowly over a period of 8–14 days so as to avoid an exacerbation of angina. However, β-blockers are contraindicated in patients with asthma, diabetes, severe bradycardia, peripheral vascular disease and chronic obstructive pulmonary disease.

18.4 Calcium Channel Blockers

18.4.1 General Description

Calcium channel blockers are commonly used in the prevention and treatment of angina pectoris, especially better for variant angina pectoris. Calcium is essential for muscular contraction. Although for the different types and chemical structure, calcium channel blockers inhibit calcium influx by blocking L-type calcium channels, which decreases contractile force and oxygen requirements. Calcium channel blockers inhibit coronary vasoconstriction or spasm; they also dilate peripheral vasculature, and decrease cardiac afterload. Their use in the treatment of exertional angina pectoris relies on the reduction in myocardial oxygen consumption resulting from decreased afterload. Their efficacy in vasospastic angina is due to the relaxation of the coronary arteries. Calcium channel blockers have a wide range of pharmacological effects and clinical applications, including antiarrhythmic effects and antihypertensive effects. Calcium channel blockers protect the tissue by inhibiting the entrance of calcium into cardiac and SMCs of the coronary and systemic arterial beds.

18.4.2 Antianginal Effects and Mechanism

1) Reduce myocardial oxygen consumption: Calcium channel blockers reduce myocardial contractility, decrease heart rate, relax vascular smooth muscle, dilate vessels, decrease blood pressure, and reduce cardiac workload, thereby reducing myocardial oxygen consumption.

2) Dilate coronary arteries: These agents relax the big transport vessels and small resistance blood vessels in the coronary artery, especially the blood vessel on spasm. Calcium channel blockers have the significant release function, thus increasing the blood perfusion in the ischemic area. In addition, calcium channel blockers increase the blood and oxygen supply in ischemic area by improving compensatory circulation.

3) Protect the ischemic myocardial cells: The permeability of cell membrane to calcium is increased in ischemia and the ability to discharge calcium from intracellular space to extracellular space is decreased. An increase in extracellular influx or a transport barrier for calcium from intracellular space to extracellular space, leads to intracellular calcium overload. Calcium channel blockers can protect myocardial cells by inhibiting the extracellular calcium influx and alleviating Ca^{2+} overload in ischemic myocardial cells. These agents also reduce the infarct size in acute myocardial infarction.

4) Inhibit platelet aggregation: Unstable angina pectoris is associated with platelet adhesion, platelet aggregation, and decreased coronary flow. Most acute myocardial infarctions are caused by the rupture of atherosclerotic plaques and the formation of thrombosis which block the coronary artery. Calcium channel blockers block the flow of calcium, decrease the concentration of calcium in platelet and inhibit platelet aggregation.

18.4.3 Therapeutic Applications

In addition to having many similarities with β-blockers in the treatment of angina pectoris, calcium channel blockers have the following advantages: ① Calcium channel blockers are more suitable for myocardial ischemia with bronchial asthma due to the relaxation of bronchial smooth muscle. ② Calcium channel blockers have a strong role in the expansion of coronary arteries; they are useful for each type of angina by coronary vasodilation, especially for variant angina. ③ Calcium channel blockers have a weak inhibitory effect on myocardial function; especially nifedipine, which has a strong peripheral vascular expansion, that can reduce peripheral resistance. The enhancement of myocardial contractility by lowering blood pressure partially counteracts the inhibitory effect on myocardium, thus reducing the risk of induction of heart failure. β-blockers are contraindicated in patients with myocardial ischemia and peripheral vascular disease, whereas calcium channel blockers are suitable for the treatment of such patients due to the expansion of peripheral blood vessels. Calcium channel blockers commonly used for angina pectoris are nifedipine, verapamil and diltiazem. These drugs are also used in cases where nitrates are ineffective or when β-blockers are contraindicated. Calcium channel antagonists should be used cautiously in combination with β-blockers, as both groups induce negative inotropic effects (i.e., depress cardiac contractility). Nifedipine may cause reflex tachycardia for hypotension action, which can exacerbate isch-

emic heart disease. Diltiazem can be given cautiously with β-blockers even though it has a lesser negative inotropic effect than verapamil.

18.4.4 Selected Drugs

18.4.4.1 Verapamil

Verapamil slows conduction through the AV node, which may be useful for angina with arrhythmia. Verapamil is not used alone in the treatment of variant angina pectoris due to the weak vasodilation of coronary artery. It is effective in the treatment of stable angina pectoris, and has a synergistic effect with β-blockers. Verapamil may produce atrioventricular block when used in combination with β-blockers, so attention should be paid to patients with systolic ventricular dysfunction, because of the additive negative effect on cardiac conduction and the high risk of heart block and severe bradycardia. Verapamil should be forbidden for angina pectoris patients with heart failure, sinus or atrioventricular node block.

18.4.4.2 Nifedipine (硝苯地平)

Nifedipine has predominant actions in the coronary artery and peripheral vasculature. Nifedipine decreases afterload and to a lesser extent preload of the heart, thereby lowering blood pressure. Nifedipine has a lesser effect on heart than verapamil. And therefore, it is particularly useful in patients with variant angina. Nifedipine is better for variant angina pectoris, especially for patients with hypertension. Nifedipine is also effective in the treatment of stable angina pectoris. It can promote the collateral circulation and reduce the infarct area in patients with acute myocardial infarction. Nifedipine and β-blockers have synergistic effect in the treatment of stable angina pectoris.

18.4.4.3 Diltiazem (地尔硫䓬)

Diltiazem, a benzodiazepine, is intermediate in properties between verapamil and nifedipine. Diltiazem is used to treat variant angina, whether naturally occurring or drug-induced, and stable angina pectoris. Diltiazem should be used with caution in patients with heart failure due to the inhibition of myocardial contractility. Diltiazem is also cautiously used to treat angina pectoris with atrioventricular block or sinus bradycardia.

18.4.5 Adverse Effects

The common adverse effects of calcium channel blockers are peripheral edema, constipation, palpitation, hypotension, facial flushing and skin rash. Other adverse effects include headache and dizziness. Calcium channel blockers may cause cardiac depression resulting from extreme inhibition of myocardial calcium influx, which can lead to bradycardia, atrioventricular block and even cardiac arrest.

Summary

心绞痛是由于心肌血氧供需失衡导致的临床综合征，降低心脏耗氧和/或增加心脏供血可以减轻心绞痛。常用的抗心绞痛药主要有硝酸酯类，β-受体阻断药和钙通道阻滞药。硝酸甘油是缓解心绞痛发作的常用药物，适用于各种类型心绞痛的治疗，为稳定型心绞痛的首选药。硝酸甘油通过释放出一氧化氮，活化鸟苷酸环化酶，使血管平滑肌细胞内cGMP生成增多，进而激活cGMP依赖性蛋白激酶，减少细胞内Ca^{2+}释放和抑制Ca^{2+}内流，使血管平滑肌松弛而产生抗心绞痛作用。β受体阻断药通过阻断β受体，减少心肌耗氧量，增加心肌缺血区的血供和氧供，改善缺血区心肌代谢，抑制血小板聚集进而发挥抗心绞痛的作用。钙通道阻滞药通过阻断心肌和血管平滑肌细胞膜上的Ca^{2+}通道，抑制细胞外Ca^{2+}内流，使细胞内Ca^{2+}水平降低，减弱心肌收缩力、扩张血管，从而降低心肌耗氧量、增加缺血区血液供应及对缺血心肌的保护作用等途径发挥其抗心绞痛的作用。

Yang Hongyan (杨宏艳)

Chapter 19   Antihypertensive Drugs

Hypertension is defined as having a sustained systolic blood pressure greater than 140mmHg or a sustained diastolic blood pressure of greater than 90mmHg. Specific etiology of hypertension can happen in only 10%–15% of patients. People without specific etiology of hypertension are said to have primary hypertension. Patients with a specific cause are said to have secondary hypertension. Hypertension is the most common cardiovascular disease. Sustained arterial hypertension damages blood vessels in kidney, heart, and brain and leads to an increased incidence of renal failure, coronary disease, heart failure, stroke, and dementia. Elevated blood pressure is usually caused by a combination of several (multifactorial) abnormalities. Epidemiologic evidence points to genetic factors, psychological stress, and environmental and dietary factors (increased salt and decreased potassium or calcium intake) as contributing to the development of hypertension.

19.1   Classification of Antihypertensive Drugs

Antihypertensive drugs (抗高血压药) are defined as the drugs that reduce blood pressure and are used to treat hypertension. Effective pharmacologic lowering of blood pressure has been shown to prevent damage to blood vessels and to substantially reduce morbidity and mortality rates. Many effective drugs are available. Knowledge of their antihypertensive mechanisms and sites of action allows accurate prediction of efficacy and toxicity. As a result, rational use of these agents, alone or in combination, can lower blood pressure with minimal risk of serious toxicity in most patients. Antihypertensive drugs are categorized according to the principal regulatory sites or mechanism. The classification is as follows:

1) **Diuretics, such as hydrochlorothiazide.**
2) **Sympathoplegic agents**
① Centrally acting sympathomimetic agents, such as clonidine.
② Adrenoceptor antagonists, such as propranolol.
③ Adrenergic neuronal blocking agents, such as reserpine.
④ Ganglionic blocking agents, such as trimethaphan camsylate.
3) **Agents that affect the RAAS**
① ACEIs, such as captopril.
② ARBs, such as losartan potassium.
③ Inhibitors of renin activity, such as aliskiren.
4) **Calcium channel blockers, such as nifedipine.**
5) **Direct vasodilators, such as hydralazine.**

19.2   Commonly Used Antihypertensive Drugs

19.2.1   Diuretics

19.2.1.1   Pharmacological effects

Diuretics lower blood pressure by depleting the body of sodium and reducing blood volume and perhaps by other mechanisms. The thiazides (噻嗪类) and the thiazide-like diuretics are generally regarded as the diuretics of choice in the management of hypertension. They are effective in lowering blood pressure by 10mmHg–15mmHg. When administered alone, thiazide diuretics can provide relief for mild or moderate hypertension.

19.2.1.2   Therapeutic Applications

Diuretics are used in combination with sympatholytic agents or vasodilators in severe hypertension. The effects of these group diuretics are more prolonged than those of the loop diuretics, the cost of therapy is low and, in combination with β-blockers, they have been shown to reduce morbidity and mortality in people with chronic hypertension. However, the precise mechanism of the antihypertensive action of the thiazides remains unclear.

19.2.1.3   Adverse Effects

When they are used to treat hypertension, the most common adverse effect of diuretics (except for potassium-sparing diuretics) is potassium depletion. Although mild degrees of hypokalemia are tolerated well by many patients, hypokalemia may be hazardous in patients taking digitalis, those who have chronic arrhythmias, or those with acute myocardial infarction or left ventricular dysfunction. Diuretics may also cause magnesium depletion, impair glucose tolerance, and increase serum lipid concentrations. Diuretics increase uric acid concentrations and may precipitate gout. The use of low doses minimizes these adverse metabolic effects without impairing the antihypertensive action. Loop diuretics are used in combination with sympatholytic agents and vasodilators for hypertension refractory to thiazide treatment. Potassium-sparing diuretics are used to avoid potassium depletion, especially when administered with cardiac glycosides.

19.2.2 Calcium Channel Blockers

Calcium channel blockers (CCBs) inhibit the entry of calcium into cardiac and smooth muscle cells by blocking the L-type Ca^{2+} channel; they lower blood pressure by reducing peripheral resistance. CCBs are effective in the treatment of mild-to-moderate hypertension. They are used for treatment of hypertension including verapamil, nifedipine, nicardipine, nisoldipine, isradipine, amlodipine, felodipine and diltiazem. Short-acting preparations of the dihydropyridines, such as nifedipine, have been associated with an increase in cardiovascular mortality and events, including MI and increased anginal attacks.

19.2.3 β-Adrenoreceptor Antagonists

Of the large number of β-blockers tested, most have been shown to be effective in lowering blood pressure. Several of these drugs have different pharmacologic properties that may confer therapeutic benefits in certain clinical situations.

19.2.3.1 Propranolol

1) **Pharmacological effects:** Propranolol is the first β-blocker shown to be effective in hypertension and ischemic heart disease. It antagonizes catecholamine action at both β_1- and β_2-receptors. Propranolol produces sustained reduction in peripheral vascular resistance. Blockade of cardiac β_1-receptors reduces heart rate and contractility. β_2-blockers increases airway resistance and decreases catecholamine induced glycogenolysis and peripheral vasodilation.

2) **Therapeutic applications:** Blockade of β-receptors in the CNS decreases sympathetic activity. Propranolol also decreases renin release. It is used in mild-to-moderate hypertension. Resting bradycardia and a reduction in the heart rate during exercise are indicators of propranolol's β-blocking effect and changes in these parameters may be used as guides for regulating dosage. Propranolol can be administered twice daily and slow-release preparations are available.

3) **Adverse effects:** The principal toxicities of propranolol result from blockade of cardiac, vascular or bronchial β-receptors. The most important of these predictable extensions of the β-blocking action occur in patients with bradycardia or cardiac conduction disease, asthma, peripheral vascular insufficiency and diabetes. When propranolol is discontinued after prolonged regular use, some patients experience a withdrawal syndrome, manifested by nervousness, tachycardia, increased intensity of angina and increased blood pressure. Although the incidence of these complications is probably low, propranolol should not be discontinued abruptly. The withdrawal syndrome may involve up-regulation or supersensitivity of β-receptors.

19.2.3.2 Metoprolol and atenolol

Metoprolol and atenolol, which are cardioselective are the most widely used β-blockers in the treatment of hypertension. Metoprolol is approximately equipotent to propranolol in inhibiting stimulation of β_1-receptors such as those in the heart but 50- to 100-fold less potent than propranolol in blocking β_2-receptors. Relative cardiac selectivity may be advantageous in treating hypertensive patients who also suffer from asthma, diabetes, or peripheral vascular disease. Although cardiac selectivity is not complete, metoprolol causes less bronchial constriction than propranolol at doses that produce equal inhibition of β_1-adrenoceptor responses. The drug has a relatively short half-life of 4-6 hours, but the extended-release preparation can be taken once daily. Sustained-release metoprolol is effective in reducing mortality from heart failure and is particularly useful in patients with hypertension and heart failure. Atenolol is not extensively metabolized and is excreted primarily in the urine with a half-life of 6 hours; it is usually dosed once daily.

19.2.4 Angiotensin Converting Enzyme Inhibitors

19.2.4.1 Pharmacological effects

Captopril and other drugs in this class inhibit the converting enzyme peptidyl dipeptidase that hydrolyzes angiotensin I to angiotensin II and inactivates bradykinin, a potent vasodilator, which works at least in part by stimulating release of nitric oxide and prostacyclin. The hypotensive activity of captopril results both from an inhibitory action on the renin-angiotensin system and a stimulating action on the kallikrein-kinin system. The latter mechanism has been demonstrated by showing that a bradykinin receptor antagonist, icatibant, blunts the blood pressure lowering effect of captopril. ACE inhibitors reduce vascular resistance and blood volume; they lower blood pressure by decreasing total peripheral resistance.

19.2.4.2 Therapeutic applications

ACE inhibitors have a particularly useful role in treating patients with chronic kidney disease because they diminish proteinuria and stabilize renal function (even in the absence of lowering of blood pressure). This effect is particularly valuable in diabetes, and these drugs are now recommended in diabetes even in the absence of hypertension. These benefits probably result from improved intrarenal hemodynamics, with decreased glomerular efferent arteriolar resistance and a resulting reduction in intraglomerular capillary pressure. They have also proved to be extremely useful in the treatment of heart failure and after myocardial infarction. There is recent evidence that ACE inhibitors reduce the incidence of diabetes in patients with high cardiovascular risk.

19.2.4.3 Adverse effects

Severe hypotension can occur after initial doses of any ACE inhibitor in patients who are hypovolemic as a result of diuretics, salt restriction, or gastrointestinal fluid loss. Other adverse effects common to all ACE inhibitors include acute renal failure, hyperkalemia, dry cough sometimes accompanied by wheezing and angioedema.

19.2.5 Angiotensin Ⅱ Receptor Blockers

Losartan and valsartan are the first marketed blockers of the angiotensin Ⅱ type 1 (AT₁) receptor. Candesartan, eprosartan, irbesartan, telmisartan, and olmesartan are also available. They have no effect on bradykinin metabolism and are therefore more selective blockers of angiotensin effects than ACE inhibitors. They also have the potential for more complete inhibition of angiotensin action compared with ACE inhibitors because there are enzymes other than ACE that are capable of generating angiotensin Ⅱ. Angiotensin receptor blockers provide benefits similar to those of ACE inhibitors in patients with heart failure and chronic kidney disease. The adverse effects are similar between them, including the hazard of use during pregnancy. Cough and angioedema can occur but are less common with angiotensin receptor blockers than with ACE inhibitors.

19.3 Other Antihypertensive Drugs

19.3.1 Centrally Acting Sympathomimetic Agents

Centrally acting sympathomimetic agents reduce peripheral resistance, inhibit cardiac function and increase pooling in capacitance venules. With the exception of clonidine, these drugs are rarely used today.

Clonidine (可乐定) stimulates postsynaptic α₂-receptors in the central nervous system (CNS) and causes reduction in total peripheral resistance. This drug is frequently combined with a diuretic and commonly produces drowsiness, lethargy, dry mouth, and constipation. Clonidine is available as a transdermal patch (Catapres-TTS) that allows weekly dosing.

19.3.2 Vasodilators

Vasodilators (血管扩张剂) relax smooth muscle and lower total peripheral resistance, thereby lowering blood pressure. The use of vasodilators is declining as a result of newer modalities, such as ACE inhibitors and calcium channel blockers, which are more effective with fewer adverse effects.

Sodium nitroprusside (硝普钠) dilates both resistance and capacitance vessels; it increases heart rate but not cardiac output. This drug is frequently used in hypertensive emergencies because of its rapid action. Sodium nitroprusside is usually administered with furosemide. On initial infusion, it may cause excessive vasodilation and hypotension. Sodium nitroprusside can be converted to cyanide and thiocyanate. The accumulation of cyanide and risk of toxicity are minimized by concomitant administration of sodium thiosulfate or hydroxocobalamin.

19.3.3 α₁-Adrenoreceptor Antagonists

α₁-Adrenoreceptor antagonists (α₁肾上腺素受体阻断剂) lower total peripheral resistance by preventing stimulation (and consequent vasoconstriction) of α-receptors, which are located predominantly in resistance vessels of the skin, mucosa, intestine, and kidney. These drugs reduce pressure by dilating resistance and conductance vessels. The effectiveness of these drugs diminishes in some patients because of tolerance.

Summary

高血压是最常见的心血管疾病。它是引起脑卒中的主要病因，高血压能够引起心肌梗死和心源性猝死等冠状动脉疾病，是导致心力衰竭、肾功能不全和主动脉夹层动脉瘤的主要原因。因此高血压治疗的主要目的是"降低高血压，保护心脑肾"，最大限度地降低心脑血管疾病的发病和死亡的总风险。

抗高血压药物是一类可降低血压，用于治疗高血压的药物。利尿剂、钙拮抗剂、β-肾上腺素受体拮抗剂、血管紧张素转换酶抑制剂和血管紧张素Ⅱ受体拮抗剂被认为是抗高血压的一线药物，除此之外，其他抗高血压药如中枢性降压药和血管扩张药等也可用于高血压的治疗。在过去十年中，开发了一些针对新靶点的药物。肾素抑制剂、5-羟色胺受体拮抗剂，前列环素合成促进剂、内皮素受体抑制剂具有潜在的治疗意义。其中一些已在临床上使用，并在治疗高血压过程中显示出特殊的优势。

降压治疗是终身疗法。应考虑逆转或预防高血压终末期器官损害。有效降低血压、降低血压变异性、阻断肾素-血管紧张素系统可能是高血压

的器官保护中最重要的环节。同时使用不同种类的药物是实现有效控制血压和减少剂量相关不良反应的常用策略。

Zhang Qi (张奇)

Chapter 20　Antiatherosclerotic Drugs

20.1　General Description

Atherosclerosis (AS) is the main cause of coronary heart disease, cerebral infarction and peripheral vascular disease. Lipid metabolism disorder as the foundation of atherosclerotic lesions, is characterized by the arterial lesions that begin with the inner membrane, general first lipid and compound carbohydrate accumulation, hemorrhage and thrombosis, and fibrous tissue hyperplasia and calcinosis, and middle artery gradual disintegration and calcification, which results in thickening of arterial wall and narrowing of vascular cavity. The lesions are usually associated with large muscular arteries, and once developed they are enough to block the artery, the tissue or organ supplied by the artery leading to ischemia or necrosis.

Atherosclerosis is caused by multiple factors, and the mechanism is complicated and has not been fully elucidated. The main risk factors include hypertension, hyperlipidemia and heavy smoking, as well as diabetes mellitus, obesity and genetic factors, and so on. The symptoms of atherosclerosis mainly depend on the blood vessel lesion and the degree of ischemia of the affected organ. There are no specific symptoms of aortic atherosclerosis; angina pectoris, myocardial infarction, arrhythmia, and evensudden death may occur in coronary atherosclerosis, if the pipe diameter of stenosis is more than 75%. Cerebral atherosclerosis can cause cerebral ischemia, cerebral atrophy, or rupture of the cerebral blood vessels. Renal atherosclerosis often leads to enuresis, refractory hypertension, even renal failure. Mesenteric atherosclerosis can be characterized by abdominal pain, indigestion, constipation, *etc.* Severe cases of intestinal wall necrosis can result in the hematochezia, paralytic ileus, etc. Severe stenosis of the vascular cavity caused by the lower limb atherosclerosis disease can lead to intermittent claudication, absent pulsation of dorsal artery of foot, even gangrene.

Atherosclerosis is treated with comprehensive methods including drug therapy and surgery. Drug therapy plays an important role in atherosclerosis. Drugs to prevent atherosclerosis include blood-lipid modulators (调血脂药), antioxidants (抗氧化剂), polyene fatty acids (多烯脂肪酸类), mucopolysaccharides (黏多糖) and polysaccharides (多糖类).

20.2　Blood-Lipid Modulators

Blood lipids (血脂) are the lipids in plasma or serum, including cholesterol (Ch, 胆固醇), triglyceride (TG, 三酰甘油), phospholipid (PL, 磷脂), and free fatty acid (FFA, 游离脂肪酸). Cholesterol is also divided into cholesterol esters (ChE, 胆固醇酯) and free cholesterol (FC, 游离胆固醇), which add up to total-cholesterol (TC, 总胆固醇). The apoproteins (Apo, 载脂蛋白) are mainly A, B, C, D and E, and they are divided into subcomponents. Different lipoproteins contain different Apo, and their main function is to combine and transport lipids. Blood lipids and apoprotein combine to form lipoprotein (LP, 脂蛋白) and then dissolve in plasma, then transport and metabolize. LP is divided into chylomicron (CM, 乳糜微粒), very low density lipoprotein (VLDL, 极低密度脂蛋白), low density lipoprotein (LDL, 低密度脂蛋白) and high density lipoprotein (HDL, 高密度脂蛋白).

Lipoprotein(a) [Lp(a), 脂蛋白(a)] is the lipoprotein that is extracted from LDL. Its physicochemical property and structure are very common with LDL. Elevated Lp(a) is an independent risk factor for atherosclerosis and is not associated with increased LDL and Ch in plasma.

All kinds of lipoproteins have basically constant concentrations in the plasma to maintain the balance between each other, and if the proportion is disordered, lipid metabolism disorder occurs, which is an important factor in atherosclerosis. Some blood lipids or lipoproteins are higher than normal and are known as hyperlipidemia or hyperlipoproteinemia (高脂蛋白血症). In order to analyze the illness and accurate medication, hyperlipoproteinemia is generally divided into six types, including Ⅰ, Ⅱ$_a$, Ⅱ$_b$, Ⅲ, Ⅳ, Ⅴ types, in which Ⅱ$_a$, Ⅱ$_b$, Ⅲ, Ⅳ types are prone to coronary heart disease.

It is generally believed that hyperlipidemia can promote the formation and development of atherosclerotic lesions. For the metabolic disorders of plasma lipids, the first step is to control diet, adjust lifestyle and avoid other cardiovascular risk factors. If lipid levels cannot be restored, blood-lipid modulators should be administrated as soon as possible according to the types of dyslipidemia, the symptoms of atherosclerosis, or other cardiovascular risk factors, to treat hyperlipoproteinemia.

20.2.1 3-hydroxy-3-methylglutaryl CoA Reductase Inhibitor

HMG-CoA reductase inhibitors are also known as statins (他汀类). HMG-CoA reductase is the rate-limiting enzyme in the process of cholesterol synthesis in hepatocytes, catalyzing HMG-CoA to generate mevalonic acid (**MVA**, 甲羟戊酸), which is the key step in the endogenous cholesterol synthesis. Inhibition of HMG-CoA reductase reduces the synthesis of endogenous cholesterol.

20.2.1.1 Pharmacological effects and mechanism

1) The effects and mechanism of regulating blood lipids: Statins have an obvious effect of regulating blood lipids. In the therapeutic dose, they exert the strongest effect to lower LDL-C whereas exert stronger effect for total cholesterd and, weak effect for triglycerides with a dose-dependent manner. It will take 2 weeks to achieve effectiveness, and 4–6 weeks to reach the peak effect. HDL-C is slightly elevated and long-term application is required to be effective.

The cholesterol in the body is mainly produced in the liver catalyzed by HMG-CoA reductase. The chemical structure of statins is similar to that of HMG-CoA. The affinity of statins for HMG-CoA reductase is thousands of times higher than that of HMG-CoA. Statins have a competitive inhibitory effect on enzymes and inhibit cholesterol synthesis. Statins not only reduce plasma cholesterol concentration, but also lead to compensatory increase of LDL receptors to reduce plasma LDL through negative feedback regulation. This leads to a fast metabolism of VLDL resulting in decreased VLDL and TG. Elevated HDL may be an indirect result of reduced VLDL. Since various statins have different affinity with HMG-CoA reductase, the effect of regulating blood lipids varies.

2) The effects of non-regulating blood lipids: It is also known as the pleiotropic effects of statins, mainly including: ① Improve the endothelial function and improve the reactivity of vascular endothelium to vasodilation; ② Inhibit the proliferation and migration of vascular smooth muscle cells (VSMCs) and promote the apoptosis of VSMCs; ③ Reduce the plasma C-reactive protein (C反应蛋白) and reduce the inflammatory response of atherosclerosis; ④ Inhibit the adhesion and secretion of mononuclear macrophages; ⑤ Antithrombotic effect is also found by inhibiting platelets aggregation and improving fibrinolytic activity; ⑥ Antioxygenation is played by scavenging oxygen-free radicals; ⑦ Reduce the formation of macrophages and foam cells in the arterial wall, which makes the atherosclerotic plaque stable and smaller.

3) Renal protection: The statins have a protective effect on kidney not only relying on lowering cholesterol, but also on anti-cell proliferation, anti-inflammation, immunosuppression, anti-osteoporosis and other functions, which can reduce the degree of renal damage.

20.2.1.2 Therapeutic applications

1) Regulating blood lipids: Statins are mainly used for heterozygous familial and non familial II_a, II_b and III type hyperlipoproteinemia, and used for hypercholesteremia (高胆固醇血症) caused by type 2 diabetes (2型糖尿病) and nephrotic syndrome (肾病综合征). In the severe cases they can be combined with bile acid-binding resins. Recently, large-scale clinical trials have shown that statins are effective and safe for both primary and secondary prevention of coronary heart disease, which can significantly reduce the morbidity and mortality of coronary heart disease.

2) Nephrotic syndrome: Statins protect and improve renal function, which may be related to the inhibition of the proliferation of glomerular membrane cells and the postponement of renal arteriosclerosis, in addition to the effect of lipids regulating.

3) Acute cardio-cerebrovascular attack: Statins can increase the stability of atheromatous plaque and reduce the plaque, thus reducing the occurrence of ischemic cerebral apoplexy, stable and unstable angina, fatal and non-fatal myocardial infarction.

4) Others: Statins can inhibit restenosis after percutaneous transluminal coronary angioplasty, alleviate the rejection reaction after organ transplantation and treat osteoporosis (骨质疏松症), and so on.

20.2.1.3 Adverse effects

A few and light adverse reactions may happen when stains are used. In large dosage, patients may have gastrointestinal reactions, muscle pain, skin flushing, headache and other temporary reactions. Occasionally, there are symptoms of elevated transaminase and creatine konase (CK, 肌酸激酶), which can be returned to normal after withdrawal. The incidence of rhabdomyolysis is higher when it is used with cerivastatin (西立伐他汀) and simvastatin, but lower with fluvastatin. Most of them are myopathy, and very few rhabdomyolysis are developed. Extra-large dosage of statins can lead to cataract in dogs, so attention should be paid to human medication. The liver function should be monitored regularly during the medication, and CK should be detected by the muscle pain. Stains should be stopped when necessary. Pregnant women, children, lactating women, patients with abnormal function of liver and kidney are not suitable for the application. Patients with a history of liver disease should be used with caution.

20.2.1.4 Statins commonly used in the clinical practice

1) Lovastatin (洛伐他汀): Lipid-regulating effect is stable and reliable in a dose-dependent manner. The effect is obvious after two weeks, and the best therapeutic effect will be obtained in 4 to 6 weeks.

2) Simvastatin (辛伐他汀): It is twice as potent as lovastatin. Its effect on elevating HDL and Apo AI is stronger than that of atorvastatin (阿伐他汀). Clinical trials show that long-term application simvastatin can regulate blood lipids as well as significantly delay atherosclerosis progression and deterioration, and reduce the occurrence of cardiac events and unstable angina.

3) Pravastatin (普伐他汀): In addition to reducing lipids, pravastatin can inhibit adhesion and aggregation of mononuclear-macrophages in the endothelium, which has anti-inflammatory effects. Studies show that it can reduce cardiovascular diseases through anti-inflammatory effects. Studies have confirmed that the early application of pravastatin in acute coronary syndromes can rapidly improve endothelial function, and reduce coronary artery stenosis and cardiovascular events.

4) Fluvastatin (氟伐他汀): Fluvastatin can block substrates as well as products of the HMG-CoA reductase at the same time, thereby inhibit MVA to produce cholesterol and regulate blood lipids. In the meantime, fluvastatin can increase NO activity, improve endothelial function, anti-vascular smooth muscle cell proliferation and prevent plaque formation. Furthermore, the drug can reduce the plasma Lp(a) level, inhibit platelet activity and improve insulin resistance.

5) Atorvastatin (阿托伐他汀): It has similar properties and indications to fluvastatin. But its effect on reducing triglycerides is stronger than that of fluvastatin. The high dose is effective for homozygous familial hypercholesterolemia.

6) Rosuvastatin (瑞舒伐他汀): It can inhibit the activity of HMG-CoA reductase and is stronger than other commonly used statins, so that inhibition on cholesterol synthesis is significantly stronger than other statins. Rosuvastatin can significantly lower the LDL-C and raise HDL-C. Lowering LDL-C is fast, and it can drop by 10% after two weeks. It is used to treat hyperlipidemia and hypercholesterolemia.

20.2.2 Nicotinic Acid

20.2.2.1 Pharmacological effects and mechanism

Nicotinic acid is one of the B vitamins, high-dose can reduce TG in the serum, prevent experimental atherosclerosis. And it has been proved that its antiatherosclerotic property is not related to the conversion of nicotinamide in vivo. If nicotinic acid and other substances are combined into esters, it is still effective to release nicotinic acid in the body. Nicotinic acid can lower TG and VLDL in the plasma, and is administered for 1 to 4 hours. Nicotinic acid can lower LDL by slow and weak process, and is administered for 5 to 7 days, and its maximum effect is achieved by 3 to 5 weeks. If nicotinic acid is used in combination with bile acid binding resins, its effect is enhanced, and if combined with statins, the effect is stronger. Nicotinic acid can raise HDL in the plasma. Nicotinic acid is recently found to be one of the few drugs to reduce Lp(a).

Nicotinic acid can reduce the level of cAMP in cells, reduce the activity of lipase, reduce decomposition of TG in adipose tissue to FFA, make raw material for hepatic TG synthesis insufficient, therefore, the synthesis and release of VLDL is reduced and the source of LDL is reduced. Nicotinic acid increases HDL, which is caused by reducing the concentration of TG, resulting in reduction of HDL metabolism. The increase of HDL is beneficial to the retrograde transport of cholesterol, preventing the development of atherosclerotic lesions. In addition, nicotinic acid can also inhibit the formation of TXA_2 and increase the formation of PGI_2, which play a role in inhibiting platelet aggregation and vasodilation.

20.2.2.2 Therapeutic applications

Nicotinic acid is a broad-spectrum blood lipid regulating drug that works best on type II_b and IV. It is applicable to mixed hyperlipidemia, hypertriglyceridemia (高甘油三酯血症), low HDL hyperlipemia, and so on. Combination with statins or fibrates can improve the curative effect.

20.2.2.3 Adverse effects

If nicotinic acid is used in large dosage, the skin flushes red, which is accompanied by itching. If used with aspirin, adverse effects can be reduced. Aspirin not only alleviates the dilatation of skin vessels caused by nicotinic acid, but also extends its half-life and prevents the increase of uric acid concentration caused by nicotinic acid. In addition, nicotinic acid can also stimulate the gastric mucosa, cause or aggravate peptic ulcer, which can be relieved after a meal. Long-term application can cause dry skin, pigmentation or acanthosis. Occasionally, abnormal liver function, increased blood uric acid, reduced glucose tolerance may appear, and can be recovered after drug withdrawal. Peptic ulcer, diabetes and liver function abnormality are contraindications.

20.2.3 Fibrates

Fibrates are derivatives of fibric acid that lower serum triacylglycerols and increase HDL levels. At present, the commonly used new types of fibrates include gemfibrazil (吉非贝齐), benzafibrate (苯扎贝特) and fenofibrate (非诺贝特), and so on.

20.2.3.1 Pharmacological effects and mechanism

Pharmacological effects of fibrates include regulating blood lipids and non-regulating blood lipids. Fibrates can reduce TG, VLDL-C, TC, and LDL-C in plasma, and raise HDL-C. But different kinds of fibrates have different strength; the effects of gemfibrazil, benzafibrate and fenofibrate are stronger. The effects of non-regulating blood lipids include anticoagulation, anti-thrombosis and anti-inflammatory, etc., which work together to exert anti-atherosclerosis effect.

Mechanism of effects may be mainly related to the activation of the nuclear receptor peroxisome proliferator-activated receptor-α (PPARα) which belongs to steroid hormone receptors, which regulate gene expression in LPL, Apo C Ⅲ, Apo AⅠ, and so on, reduce the transcription of Apo CⅢ, increase the generation and activity of LPL and Apo AⅠ, at the same time, promote the uptake of fatty acids in the liver, and inhibit the synthesis of TG, reduce lipoproteins that contain TG. The activation of the PPAR-α can increase the activity of inducible nitric oxide synthase (iNOS, 诱导型一氧化氮合酶), which makes NO increase, thus inhibiting expression of matrix metalloproteinase-9 (MMP-9) in macrophages. It is associated with atherosclerotic plaques stability. PPARα is also a kind of inflammatory adjustment factor. Activated PPAR-α can not only regulate blood lipids, but also reduce the inflammatory reaction in the process of atherosclerosis, inhibit vascular smooth muscle cell proliferation and restenosis after percutaneous transluminal coronary angioplasty. In addition, the fibrates have the effects of non-regulating blood lipids, such as reducing the activity of certain clotting factors and reducing the production of plasminogen activator inhibitor (PAI-1, 纤溶酶原激活物抑制物).

20.2.3.2 Therapeutic applications

Fibrates mainly are used for primary hypertriglyceridemia, also have good curative effect on type Ⅲ hyperlipoproteinemia and mixed hyperlipoproteinemia. They can also be used for the hyperlipoproteinemia of type Ⅱ diabetes.

20.2.3.3 Adverse effects

The adverse effects of fibrates are mainly gastrointestinal reactions, such as loss of appetite, nausea and abdominal distension, and so on. Fatigue, headache, insomnia, rash, impotence can be seen also. Occasionally, muscle pain, increase of urea nitrogen and transaminase may occur and can be restored after drug withdrawal. The adverse effects of clofibrate (氯贝丁酯) are more and more serious, which can cause arrhythmia, cholecystitis and gallstones, even increase the incidence of gastrointestinal tumor. Fibrates can enhance the anticoagulant activity of oral anticoagulants. Combined application with statins may increase the incidence of myopathy. Patients with hepatobiliary disease, pregnant women, children and renal insufficiency are prohibited to use them.

20.2.3.4 Fibrates commonly used in the clinical practice

1) Gemfibrazil: Gemfibrazil can quickly and steadily reduce TG and VLDL in plasma. It has the best effect on hyperlipidemia in which plasma TG significantly increases with HDL lowering or LDL increasing. Long-term application can significantly reduce the mortality of coronary heart disease.

2) Fenofibrate: In addition to lipid-regulating effects, fenofibrate can significantly reduce levels of plasma fibrinogen and serum uric acid, reduce plasma viscosity and improve haemodynamics. Coronary angiography has shown that it can prevent the narrowing of the coronary arteries.

3) Benzafibrate: The pharmacological effects and therapeutic applications are the same as gemfibrozil. Benzafibrate is used in type 2 diabetes with elevated blood lipids. It can reduce fasting blood glucose in addition to lipid-regulating effects. It reduces the plasma free fatty acid (FFA), fibrinogen, and glycosylated hemoglobin levels, and inhibits platelet aggregation. Long-term application can reduce the level of Lp(a) in plasma.

20.2.4 Bile Acid-binding Resin

Bile acid-binding resins mainly include the cholestyramine (考来烯胺) and colestipol (考来替泊). They are not absorbed into the intestines and are combined strongly with bile acids to block enterohepatic circulation and recycle of bile acids, thus depleting cholesterol and lowering the levels of TC and LDL-C in plasma.

20.2.4.1 Pharmacological effects and mechanism of effects

Cholestyramine is combined with bile acids through ion exchange in the intestines, and has the following effects: ① Combine bile acids and make them lose their activity, and reduce the absorption of lipids (including cholesterol) in food; ② Prevent bile acids from reabsorption in the intestines; ③ Transform hepatic cholesterol into bile acids through 7-α hydroxylase due to the loss of bile acids; ④ Because of the reduction of cholesterol in liver cells, the number or activity of LDL receptors is enhanced on the surface of liver cells; ⑤ The LDL-C enter the liver cells through the receptors, which lower the levels of TC and LDL-C in plasma; ⑥ In this process, the secondary activity of HMG-CoA reductase can be increased, but it cannot compensate for the reduction of cholesterol. If combined with statins, it has synergistic effects.

Cholestyramine can reduce the TC and LDL-C, and its intensity is related to the dose. It also reduces Apo B, but hardly affects HDL, and has little effect on TG and VLDL.

20.2.4.2　Therapeutic applications

Cholestyramine is applicable to type II_a, type II_b and familial heterozygote hyperlipoproteinemia, but it is invalid for the homozygous familial hypercholesterolemia. For II_b type hyperlipoproteinemia, it should be combined with drugs that reduce TG and VLDL.

20.2.4.3　Adverse effects

High doses of cholestyramine cause a special odor and a certain irritation. In a few cases constipation, abdominal distention, belching and loss of appetite, *etc* may occur, but generally disappear after two weeks. Occasionally, the temporary rise of transaminase, perchloric acid or fat diarrhea may occur.

20.3　Antioxidants

Oxygen free radicals play an important role in the occurrence and development of atherosclerosis. It has been proved that oxidation of LDL (ox-LDL) influences the occurrence and development process of atherosclerotic lesions, such as: ① Damage vascular endothelium, promote the adhesion of monocytes to endothelium and subcutaneous metastasis; ② Block the macrophages that are transformed by subcutaneous monocytes returning to the bloodstream; ③ Macrophages can take an unlimited amount of ox-LDL and become foam cells; ④ Promote endothelial cells to release the platelet derived growth factor (PDGF, 血小板衍生生长因子) and other substances, which lead to the proliferation and migration of vascular smooth muscle cells (VSMCs); ⑤ The lipids accumulation of foam cells forms lipid streaks and plaques; ⑥ Endothelial cells damage can also cause platelet aggregation and thrombosis. Studies have shown that Lp(a) and VLDL can also be enhanced by oxidation, leading to atherosclerosis; HDL has an anti-atherosclerotic effect and can also be oxidized and converted to the cause of atherosclerosis. Therefore, preventing oxidative modification of lipoproteins by oxygen free radicals has become an important measure to prevent the occurrence and development of atherosclerosis. The typical representative of these drugs is **probucol** (普罗布考).

20.3.1　Pharmacological Effects and Mechanism

20.3.1.1　Antioxidant effect

Probucol can inhibit the generation of ox-LDL and a series of pathological changes, such as endothelial cells damage, and proliferation and migration of VSMCs, etc.

20.3.1.2　Effect of regulating blood lipids

Probucol can decrease TC and LDL-C in plasma.

Meanwhile, HDL-C and Apo AI are significantly reduced, with no effect on plasma TG and VLDL generally. If combined with statins or bile acid-binding resins, lipid-regulating effect can be emphasized.

20.3.1.3　Effect of atherosclerotic lesions

Long-term application of probucol can reduce the incidence of coronary heart disease, stop the development or retreat of the atherosclerotic lesions that have been formed, and obviously reduce or eliminate xanthomas.

Probucol is a hydrophobic antioxidant with strong antioxidant effect, which is distributed to all the lipoproteins in the body. It is itself oxidized as a probucol radical, can block lipids peroxidation, reduce generation of lipid hydroperoxide (**LPO**, 脂质过氧化物), and slow down the process of atherosclerotic lesions. At the same time probucol can inhibit HMG-CoA reductase, reduce cholesterol synthesis, and increase the removal of LDL by receptor-mediated and non-receptor pathway, and decrease the level of LDL-C in plasma. By raising the plasma concentrations of cholesterol ester transfer protein and Apo E, it reduces cholesterol in HDL particles, raises the number and activity of HDL, increases transport efficiency of HDL, and makes the reverse transport clearance of cholesterol faster.

Anti-atherosclerotic properties of probucol may be an integrated result of antioxidation and lipid-regulating effects.

20.3.2　Therapeutic Applications

Probucol can be used for various types of hypercholesterolemia, including homozygous and heterozygous familial hypercholesterolemia. It is also effective for lipoproteinaemia type II secondary to nephrotic syndrome or diabetes. Long-term usage can cause the xanthoma (黄色瘤) to subside, block development of atherosclerotic lesions or promote regression of lesion, reduce the incidence of coronary heart disease. Probucol can prevent restenosis after PTCA.

20.3.3　Adverse Effects

Adverse effects are rare and light, mainly including gastrointestinal reactions, such as diarrhea, abdominal distension, abdominal pain, nausea, etc. Eosinophils increase, abnormal liver function, hyperuricemia, hyperglycemia, thrombocytopenia, myopathy, and paresthesia, etc. occasionally occur. Those with recent myocardial damage, pregnant women and children are prohibited to use it.

20.4　Polyene Fatty Acids

The representative of polyene fatty acids are eicosapentaenoic acid (EPA, 二十碳五烯酸) and docosahexaenoic acid (DHA, 二十二碳六烯酸).

20.4.1 Pharmacological Effects and Mechanism

EPA and DHA are mainly from marine organisms. Epidemiological survey found that the incidence of cardiovascular disease was lower in the Greenland Eskimo, mainly related to their consumption of marine animals such as sea fish. It is confirmed that these animal oils are rich in polyene fatty acids which can regulate blood lipids and have anti-atherosclerotic effects.

20.4.1.1 Effect of regulating blood lipids

EPA and DHA can obviously regulate blood lipids, lower TG and VLDL-TG, increase HDL-C. They obviously increase HDL_2 and the ratio of Apo A I / Apo A II. DHA can lower TC and LDL-C, while EPA is weak. The effect of regulating blood lipids in EPA and DHA may be associated with inhibiting the synthesis of TG and Apo B in the liver and increasing LPL activity to promote VLDL decomposition.

20.4.1.2 Effect of non-regulating blood lipids

EPA and DHA can replace the arachidonic acid (AA, 花生四烯酸), as 3-series prostaglandins (前列腺素) and 5-series leukotrienes (白三烯) precursors playing the following roles: ① Replace the AA to form TXA_3, abate the effects on promoting platelet aggregation and shrinking blood vessels of TXA_2; form PGI_3 in the blood vessel wall, which can expand blood vessels and preventplatelet aggregation as PGI_2. Therefore, antiplatelet aggregation, antithrombosis and vasodilatation are stronger. ② The effect of antiplatelets can inhibit the release of PDGF, thereby inhibiting proliferation and migration of VSMCs. ③ EPA and DHA on red cell membranes can increase the plasticity of red blood cells and improve microcirculation. ④ The EPA in the white blood cells can be converted into 5-series leukotriene such as LTB5, which attenuate 4-series leukotriene such as LTB4 promoting the adhesion and transformation of white blood cells to vascular endothelium. And the EPA can reduce the concentration of IL-1β and TNF in blood and inhibit the activity of adhesion molecule. EPA and DHA show a significant inhibitory effect on the expression of various cytokines in the leukocyte-endothelial inflammatory response during early atherosclerosis.

20.4.2 Therapeutic Applications

EPA and DHA are applicable to high TG hyperlipidemia. The prognosis of patients with myocardial infarction can be significantly improved. It can also be used for diabetes mellitus with hyperlipidemia.

20.4.3 Adverse Effects

Generally there are no adverse effects, but long-term or large dose application can prolong bleeding time and reduce immune response.

20.5 Mucopolysaccharides and Polysaccharides

Mucopolysaccharides are long chains consisting of repetitious disaccharide units which are composed of hexosamine or its derivatives and uronic acid. The typical representative is heparin. Heparin plays the role of anti-atherosclerosis in many aspects: ① Reduce TC, LDL, TG, VLDL and raise HDL. ② It has a high affinity for artery endothelium, and neutralizes various vascular active substances to protect the artery endothelium. ③ Inhibits the anti-inflammatory response of leukocytes to endothelial adhesion and subcutaneous metastasis. ④ Blocks the proliferation and migration of VSMCs. ⑤ Strengthen the microangiogenesis of acid fibroblast growth factor (aFGF, 酸性成纤维细胞生长因子). ⑥ Antithrombotic formation and so on. It is inconvenient to use because of the strong effect of anticoagulation, and low oral effect. Therefore, people have studied low molecular weight heparin and heparinoids (类肝素) which inhibit atherosclerosis as heparin without side effects on anti-atherosclerosis.

The low molecular weight heparin (**LMWH**) is formed by the depolymerization of heparin, and the average molecular weight is 4kDa to 6kDa. There are more than 10 kinds of LMWH products, such as enoxaparin (依诺肝素), tedelparin (替地肝素), fraxiparin (弗希肝素), logiparin (洛吉肝素) and lomoparin (洛莫肝素). They are mainly used for unstable angina pectoris, acute myocardial infarction and restenosis after PTCA.

Natural heparinoid are substances that exist in the organism, which is similar to heparin structure, such as heparan sulfate (硫酸乙酰肝素), dermatan sulfate (硫酸皮肤素), chondroitin sulfate (硫酸软骨素), and Guanxinshu (冠心舒). Guanxinshu is a complex of heparan sulfate, dermatan sulfate and chondroitin sulfate, derived from pig intestinal mucosa. It can regulate blood lipids, reduce myocardial oxygen consumption, inhibit platelet aggregation, protect vascular endothelium and prevent formation of atherosclerotic plaques. It is used in heart and cerebral ischemic diseases. Studies have shown that Guanxinshu has inhibitory effect on the proliferation of VSMCs with the same strength as heparin, while anticoagulation is only 1/47 of the heparin, and is effective orally, which show that natural heparinoids may be promising anti-atherosclerotic drugs.

Summary

动脉粥样硬化是一种慢性炎症过程，是心、脑血管病的主要病理学基础。因此，防治动脉粥样硬化是防治心脑血管疾病的重要措施。

动脉粥样硬化是多因素共同作用引起的，发病机制复杂，目前尚未完全阐明。各种脂蛋白在血浆中有基本恒定的浓度以维持相互之间的平衡，如果比例失调则脂代谢失常或紊乱，是引起动脉粥样硬化的重要因素。某些血脂或脂蛋白高于正常范围则称为高脂血症或高脂蛋白血症。

　　动脉粥样硬化的治疗方式有综合治疗、药物治疗和手术治疗。药物治疗在抗动脉粥样硬化方面发挥了重要作用。防治动脉粥样硬化的药物包括：调血脂药、抗氧化剂、多烯脂肪酸类、黏多糖和多糖类等。它们通过调血脂和非调血脂作用来调整血脂或脂蛋白紊乱，从而防治各种类型的高脂血症。

Wang Xiaoli（王晓丽）

参 考 文 献
REFERENCES

柏树令, 应大君, 2013. 系统解剖学. 8版. 北京: 人民卫生出版社

傅国辉, 于金德, 2010. 心血管系统. 上海: 上海交通大学出版社

李玉林, 2013. 病理学. 8版. 北京: 人民卫生出版社

刘执玉, 2009. 系统解剖学(双语版)[M]. 北京: 科学出版社

刘执玉, 应大君, 2013. 系统解剖学(双语版). 2版. 北京: 科学出版社

孙保存, 2013. 病理学. 2版. 北京: 北京大学医学出版社

唐军民, 2011. 组织学与胚胎学(双语版). 2版. 北京: 北京大学医学出版社

唐军民, 2013. 组织学与胚胎学. 3版. 北京: 北京大学医学出版社

王建枝, 陈国强, 2017. 病理生理学(双语版). 英文改编版. 北京: 科学出版社

王建枝, 金惠铭, 2007. 病理生理学(英文版). 北京: 人民卫生出版社

杨宝峰, 2013. 药理学. 8版. 北京: 人民卫生出版社

臧伟进, 吴立玲, 2015. 心血管系统. 北京: 人民卫生出版社

周庚寅, 姜叙诚. 2007. 病理学. 北京: 科学出版社

周宏灏, 2014. 药理学(双语版). 北京: 科学出版社

Bouki, et al, 2005. Management of cardiogenic shock due to acute coronary syndromes. Angiology, 56(2): 123–130

Buja L M, 2005. Netters Illustrated Human Pathology. Rochester: Saunders

Harvey R A, 2012. Pharmacology. 5th ed. Philadelphia: Lippincott Williams & Wilkins

Katz A M, 2010. Physiology of the Heart. 5st ed. Philadelphia: Lippincott Williams and Wilkins

Katzung et al, 2012. Basic & Clinical Pharmacology. 12th ed. New York: The McGraw-Hill Companies

Liang Li, 2015. Pathology. 北京: 高等教育出版社

Mcphee, et al, 2003. Pathophysiology of disease: an introduction to clinical medicine. 4th ed. Philadelphia: McGraw-Hill Company

Singh I, 1997. Textbook of Human Histology. 3rd ed. Rohtak: Lordson Publishers (P) Ltd

Standring S, 2015. Gray's Anatomy-The Anatomical Basis of Clinical Practice. 41st ed. New York: Elsevier Publishing Company

Willam F G, 2003. Cardiovascular Disorders: Vascular Disease. In: McPhee SJ, Lingappa VR and Ganong WF. Pathophysiology of disease: An introduction to clinical medicine. 4th ed. New York: McGraw-Hill Companies: 444–501